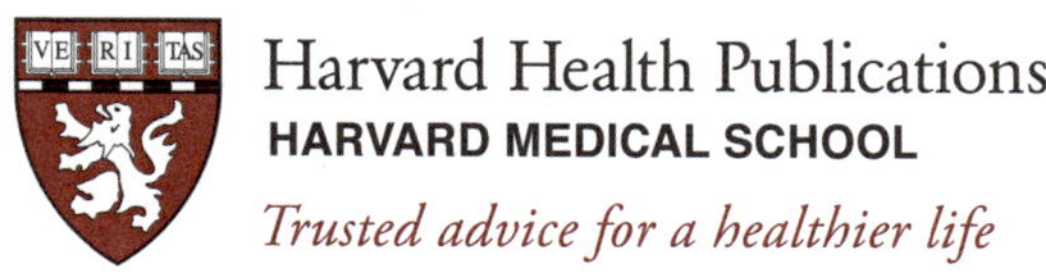

Dear Reader,

The death of someone close to you can be a transformational moment. People often define themselves in terms of their relationships: A woman may think of herself as a daughter, wife, mother, sister, or friend. A man might define himself as a brother, husband, father, son, or friend. When someone close dies, the very definition of self changes. How can you be a husband without a wife? A daughter without parents? A friend if your closest friend is gone?

Sooner or later, everyone will grieve the loss of a relative or friend, whether the cause is a sudden heart attack, a car accident, a lengthy illness, or old age. Each year, 2.4 million men, women, and children die in the United States, leaving behind many others who mourn them.

The death of someone close to you begins a process that, while painful, is a normal and expected part of the life cycle. It's an experience through which you gradually come to terms with the loss of your loved one and begin to regroup and see yourself in a new way. We hold on—in memory, and through pictures and stories—to the person who is gone, and we move on. It's common to feel overwhelmed at first by the depth and intensity of your loss. Immediately after a death, you may be plunged into funeral preparations and logistics, which distract you from having to fully register your loss and what it means to you. Over time, the reality sets in that your loved one won't return and won't be part of your daily life or your special moments, and intense loneliness and sorrow come. Most people find their way out of this dark place, with help from family and friends, and emerge into a changed, impoverished, but livable world. Supportive friends and family, good luck, time, and a sense of purpose can help mitigate the loss, but, for most people, some elements of grief persist forever.

Accepting that there is no "right" way to grieve can be a powerful first step. Doing so gives you permission to grieve at your own pace and in your own way. This Special Health Report is intended to help you do this. The report contains practical ideas based on current research and common sense. As you'll see, certain axioms about grief are backed by little or no actual evidence. Contrary to popular perception, for example, denial can be helpful. Anger isn't always part of grieving. And no single pathway leads out of grief or ensures closure. But it may help to know that most people are resilient. Often, the embrace of family, friends, and surrounding community softens sorrow. Over time, healing occurs.

Sincerely,

Susan D. Block, M.D.
Medical Editor

Harvard Health Publications | Harvard Medical School | 4 Blackfan Circle, 4th Floor | Boston, MA 02115

Understanding the grieving process

Your world has just been turned upside down. You've lost a loved one—someone so close to your heart, so much a part of the inner fabric of your life, that you feel you can't go on.

Losing someone for whom you care deeply is perhaps the most painful transition you face in life. Often, this experience is not a solitary one. The ripple effect of grief may extend to your children, your grandchildren, and everyone whose lives your loved one touched. In many cases, you are left to come to terms not only with your own sense of loss, but that of your family and friends as well.

And yet, one thing is clear: For all the pain and sorrow the death of a loved one evokes, people are remarkably resilient. Life *does* go on, if in a different way than before. It may be of some comfort to know that there is help available on this journey. Those who have walked the same path, as well as counselors who have helped guide people in times of loss, can be a source of consolation and healing.

In this report, we share some of their wisdom and suggest resources and practices to help guide you through the process, from caring for yourself to finding ways to honor your loved one. We also explore how the loss may affect family members and how they, in turn, may influence your process of mourning.

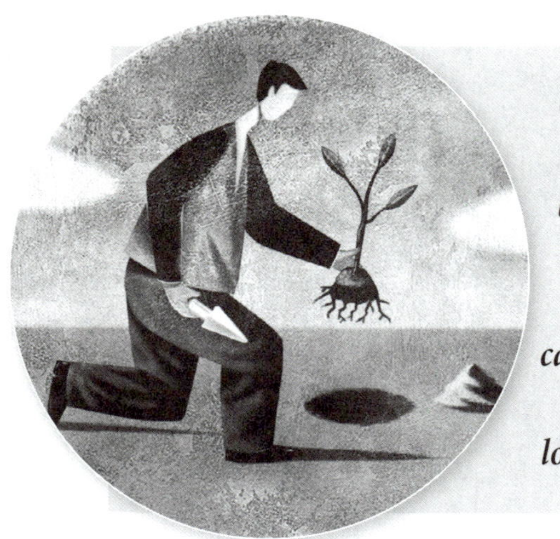

Observing rituals or paying tribute by planting a tree or holding an annual service can help mark and acknowledge the loss of a loved one.

Grief's far-reaching effects

Grief can affect both the mind and the body in dramatic ways. In a study of 33 recent widowers, researchers at Brandeis University were struck by the men's poignant, emotion-filled metaphors of loss: "I feel I am in a long dark tunnel and have not found an exit yet." "It was like a tsunami,… like an enormous wave that crashes on your family and leaves you in a sea of silence." "It's like a hole that rips through your soul."

At first, grief may permeate everything. You may find it hard to eat or sleep. It may be difficult to muster much interest in the life going on around you. You may experience restlessness, memory impairment, or difficulty concentrating. If you use alcohol, tobacco, or sedatives, you may find your consumption increasing. Symptoms similar to those the deceased had described may crop up in your own body—a frightening experience if he or she died from an illness. Some people, particularly children, may have other physical complaints, such as headaches, stomachaches, dizziness, or a racing heart.

The emotional maelstrom that grief stirs up can affect behavior and judgment. It's common, for example, to feel agitated or exhausted or to cry or withdraw from the world at times. Sometimes intrusive or upsetting memories surface, as can temporary sensations of things being unreal. In her memoir, *The Year of Magical Thinking*, author Joan Didion eloquently described her altered sense of reality after the unexpected death of her husband, the novelist and screenwriter John Gregory Dunne, and the simultaneous illness (and subsequent death) of their daughter, Quintana. She wrote:

> *There had been occasions on which I was incapable of thinking rationally. I was thinking as small children think, as if my thoughts or wishes had the power to reverse the narrative, change the outcome. In my case this disordered thinking had been covert, noticed I think by no one else, hidden even from me, but it had also been, in retrospect, both urgent and constant.*

People who are grieving regularly have the experience of sensing the presence or hearing the voice of the deceased. These experiences are not pathological. Frequent thoughts of the person who died and feelings of self-reproach about aspects of the death are normal, too.

The effects are not just emotional. You may also be more susceptible to physical illness. Among other things, studies have shown that immune cell function falls and inflammatory responses rise in people suffering bereavement. That may help explain why people often note a surge in ailments such as colds and why they tend to use more health care resources during this period. Following a loss, people are also at increased risk of hospitalization, high blood pressure (hypertension), and heart disease, and their existing medical conditions, such as heart failure, tend to worsen. Over all, they report reduced quality of life over the ensuing one to two years. Indeed, bereavement increases the risk of death from a variety of causes, including suicide. There is even an increased risk of cancer for those who develop complicated grief (see "Depression and complicated grief," below).

Expect that while you are grieving, you will not be yourself. But also know that the pain will not always be so intense. Self-care, which includes allowing yourself to be cared for, is important during these difficult times. This report offers many ideas for how to cope during this stressful time.

Depression and complicated grief

The vast majority of people who experience a loss are able to recover on their own. That's not to say that the process is easy. After the death of a close friend or family member, many people report trouble sleeping and eating, little interest in daily routines, tearful outbursts, sadness, and irritability or anger. All of these symptoms can be signs of depression or simply part of healthy grieving.

But sadness and waves of intense emotion—normal parts of the grieving process—are different from sinking into a clinical depression. Talk with your doctor or a mental health professional if you experience any of these other symptoms of bereavement-related depression:

- suicidal thoughts
- persistent feelings of worthlessness, which are common with depression but not with healthy grief
- hopelessness, helplessness
- ongoing guilt
- marked mental and physical sluggishness
- persistent trouble functioning
- hallucinations, other than occasionally thinking you hear or see the deceased.

Up to 50% of widows and widowers have symptoms typical of major depression during the first few months after a spouse's death. However, a review of studies on the topic noted that just 10% of bereaved people are depressed at the one-year mark. By two years, this dwindles to 7%. Depression can be helped with medication (antidepressants and anti-anxiety agents) and psychotherapy. A personal or family history of depression may put you at greater risk of major depression when bereaved.

If months or even years go by with no improvement, however slow or painful, you may be suffering from complicated grief or prolonged grief, which affects about 10% of the bereaved. The most common feature of complicated grief is intense, unremitting yearning and longing for the loved one. By definition, complicated grief also includes at least four of the symptoms below:

- difficulty moving on
- numbness or detachment
- bitterness
- feelings that life is empty without the deceased
- trouble accepting the death
- a sense that the future holds no meaning without the deceased
- being on edge or agitated
- difficulty trusting others since the loss
- social withdrawal
- difficulty re-engaging with life.

Talk to your doctor or a mental health professional if you experience any combination of these symptoms. Other reasons to seek professional help include drug abuse or increased use of tobacco or alcohol, suffering several losses, gaining or losing a significant amount of weight, experiencing uncontrollable anxiety, and failing to feel somewhat better after a year has passed.

How long does grief last?

Grief is not a mountain to be climbed and then descended with a map in hand. Its boundary lines differ greatly from one person to another and from one culture to the next. Americans often labor under cultural injunctions to attain "closure" within months, or certainly by the time a year has passed. Popular culture also promotes the misconception that there is an orderly progression of emotions that will lead the bereaved person to this end. The truth, though, is that grief doesn't neatly conclude at the six-month or one-year mark—even if a person follows every prescription for healthy grieving—and there is no single way to grieve. Each person has a different experience. Depending on the strength of the bond that was broken, grief can be lifelong. Often, parents whose children die say they never get over the loss. Usually, though, grief softens and changes over time.

The more integral someone was to your life, the more opportunities there are for happy and sad reminders that underscore your loss. Indeed, the death of a spouse ranks first among life events that create stress and require social readjustment. Alongside warm or warring memories, you may always carry a hollow spot in your heart. Feelings of sadness, abandonment, loss, and even anger are especially likely around birthdays, weddings, the anniversary of the death, and holidays or other occasions you might have shared. A familiar scent, song, or likeness can trigger feelings of grief, too. All of this is entirely normal.

It's also normal for the raw, all-consuming shock of early grief to ebb slowly within weeks or months, sometimes years. Gradually, at their own pace, most people do find themselves adjusting to their loss and slipping back into the routines and pleasures of daily life.

The legacy of grief is individual, multifaceted, and varied. In the midst of loss, many people find opportunities for growth. In many cases, people emerge from the depths of their grief with greater confidence in their ability to manage life's sorrows and difficulties. People often redefine themselves in terms of their position in the family or their role in the world. A death of a spouse may require the remaining spouse to become more independent and assertive, while the death of a parent may spur an adult child to assume a leadership role in the family. For some, the experience leaves them more understanding of and empathetic to other people's hardships. Losing someone close may also deepen or renew spirituality and can leave individuals with a greater appreciation of family, friends, and the pleasures of life.

One goal of this report is to describe ways for you to comfort yourself that encourage gradual acceptance of the changes in your life. You can make healing choices. You can tap into strengths you may not have realized you had (see "Draw on earlier coping skills," at left). And you can honor the person who died and the importance of your relationship in many ways. (For detailed suggestions, see "Coping with grief and loss," page 13.)

Drawing on earlier coping skills

Most people have experienced some difficulties in life, whether personal, professional, or financial. In your time of grieving, make use of what you learned from those experiences, especially those from other losses. This can help you separate approaches that don't serve you well from those that are healthy and useful.

Examine your life. A few simple questions can help you identify your coping strategies. What makes you feel better when you feel awful? What do you tend to do when you are distressed? Which of your coping strategies are helpful, and which might be hurtful?

Think back. How were deaths and losses handled in your family? Were they largely shuffled away behind closed doors or openly marked and mourned? When did you first experience the death of someone you loved? How old were you? How were you told about it? Were you allowed to participate in services? How safe was it to express your own feelings of loss? Was your grief acknowledged, or were you told implicitly or explicitly to stop being so upset? How were sad or angry feelings expressed in your family?

Replace an unhealthy approach. Try to replace one unhealthy coping strategy with a healthier possibility. For example, when you feel overwhelmed, call a friend to talk rather than downing a pint of ice cream or a stiff drink. Be judicious, though. Seeking solitude when you need it or occasionally taking second helpings of comfort food or a single drink should not necessarily be considered a problem.

Are there stages of grief?

There are many emotions that are common in bereavement. But whether these emotions occur in a standard sequence is subject to much debate. What is clear is that, as deep and permanent as your grief may seem at first, it will change over time.

A frequently cited model of bereavement, the "five stages of grief," was originally described in the 1969 book *On Death and Dying* by Elisabeth Kübler-Ross. It's worth noting that she did not intend the stages to describe bereavement, but rather the five-step response of people with serious illnesses to awareness of their impending death: denial, anger, bargaining, depression, and acceptance. The five-stage theory was later altered and adapted to cover many forms of loss, from divorce to the death of a loved one, with the five stages being disbelief, yearning, anger, depression, and acceptance. A number of researchers have found that the five stages of loss do peak in sequence, although there may be periods when the stages overlap.

Other experts frame these ideas differently, but the concept of a progression from disbelief, through emotional pain, toward acceptance, which generates the capacity to create a new life, is common to most theories. Of course, the grief process is affected by many other factors: how the person died, the quality of your relationship with him or her, and cultural, social, and economic issues.

Despite its familiar pattern, many who have experienced the grief trajectory describe it as a decidedly nonlinear experience. Grief is a stealth predator that can appear intermittently and unexpectedly. Author Joan Didion described this onslaught of emotions as "waves, paroxysms, sudden apprehensions that weaken the knees and blind the eyes and obliterate the dailiness of life."

To Facebook executive Sheryl Sandberg, whose husband died suddenly while they were on vacation in Mexico, the grief was initially overwhelming. "In those early days and weeks and months, it was always there, not just below the surface but on the surface. Simmering, lingering, festering," she writes in her 2017 book *Option B: Facing Adversity, Building Resilience, and Finding Joy*. "Then, like a wave, it would rise up and pulse through me, as if it were going to tear my heart right out of my body." Over time, however, she found that "the fog of intense pain lifted now and then, and when it rolled back in, I recovered faster." Still, her grief did not progress neatly from disbelief to acceptance. Instead, the emotions associated with the various stages seemed to rise and fall at unpredictable times. "Grief and anger aren't extinguished like flames doused with water," she writes. "They can flicker away one moment and burn hot the next."

The authors of popular books on grief prescribe various antidotes for facing this sometimes sudden onset of grief. Some offer comfort through prayers or poetic reflections. Others present step-by-step blueprints for resolution. However, grief is not a tidy, orderly process, and there is no single "right" way to grieve. New losses and joys occur. Anniversaries arrive. Understand that your ability to move ahead with your life will ebb and flow. Expect your emotions to collide and overlap. Grieve at the pace and in the way that feels right to you.

Managing denial

Often it's easier to recognize denial in others than in ourselves. If you think denial might be interfering with the grieving process of someone you care about—or if denial is hobbling your ability to move forward—the following suggestions may prove helpful. Remember, though, to be patient with the grieving person or yourself and understand that denial can be protective and useful.

Acknowledge it. Sometimes denial offers a safe haven or a much-needed break. Avoidance has a place in grief. Some bereavement experts note that when you're ready to learn more, explore more, or do more, you will. Sometimes accepting rather than pushing against denial allows other feelings to surface.

Explore it. Think about what your "stuckness" or disbelief might be protecting you from. Often, fear—of forgetting your loved one, of moving on, or of feeling overwhelming pain—is holding you back. Realizing this can help you feel more in control. Writing out your feelings may help you move forward.

If you can't seem to shake persistent numbness or a sense of disbelief, consider seeking help.

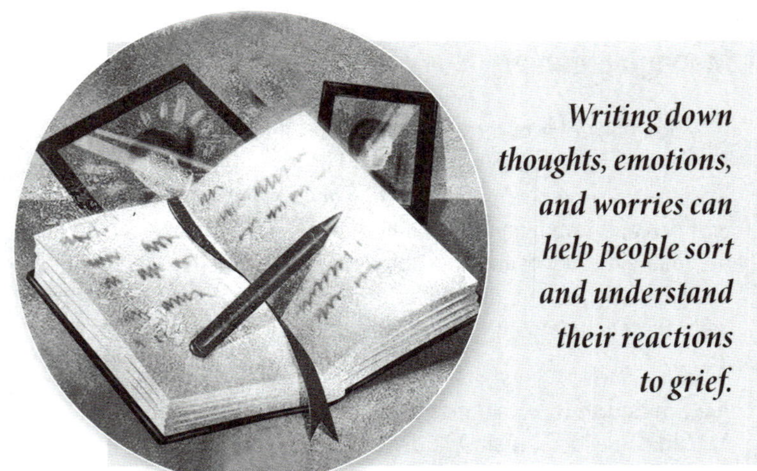

Writing down thoughts, emotions, and worries can help people sort and understand their reactions to grief.

How earlier losses shape grief

How you react to the loss of someone you love can be colored by previous painful losses in your life, including earlier deaths, job loss, divorce, disabling injury, or even the loss of a community of friends or family after moving to a new location. Unresolved or unacknowledged losses exert their influence on how you react to a new loss. Often, the losses that have the greatest impact occur during childhood. If any of these are left unaddressed, they can exaggerate your response to losses later in life. In a sense, later losses expand upon the earlier ones, building a larger and larger wall of grief to cope with.

Whatever losses you have suffered, you probably developed some type of psychological defense strategies to help you cope. Whether wielded as conscious coping tools or buried deeply in the psyche, defenses help people tolerate overwhelming anxiety and emotional pain. For example, a daughter might handle the loss of her father and its ensuing grief by developing a cheerful front that really represents a way of avoiding and denying the terrible sorrow she is experiencing. Because she does not deal with her emotional pain, but rather buries it, she becomes especially vulnerable to a later loss that overwhelms her defenses and requires her to deal with her earlier loss and the recent loss all at once.

Defenses aren't good or bad by definition, although some are more helpful and healthy than others. There is a marked difference between having several drinks every night to calm yourself and using exercise and stress-relief techniques to do the same. Likewise, long periods of social withdrawal may ease the pain of a loss, but they can also feed feelings of loneliness and depression.

Denial, anger, and guilt

Tears and sadness during bereavement are normal. People may expect you to pass through these emotions too quickly, but generally they find this behavior acceptable. Yet other emotions sparked by bereavement make many people uneasy. Chief among these are denial, anger, and guilt, which may emerge in response to a death or during the course of a terminal illness. Not everyone will feel these emotions, but many people do.

A sense of disbelief

Denial is insistence that a diagnosis of illness or a

Coping with anger

If the death of someone you love has left you feeling angry or bitter, you might find it helpful to try the following techniques.

Consider it. Is anger a stand-in for more painful emotions, or does the situation warrant it? Do you feel afraid or abandoned—by others, by God, or by the loved one who died? If so, could you enlist support from others or spend some time thinking about your distress and understanding it better? It might help to share your feelings with a spiritual leader or with members of a grief support group, who can tell how they have dealt with similar feelings.

Express it. Set aside a safe time and place each day to defuse angry feelings. Some people yell in the car with the windows rolled up. Some find stress-relief techniques like meditation or yoga helpful. Others find release in punching pillows or in exercise. Think about options for releasing anger, and plan how to express it safely when it crops up. Sometimes writing about situations that make you feel angry can help you focus on what you are really feeling beneath your anger.

Explain it. Tell others how short-fused you are right now. If you know you stepped over the line, apologize. Most people will make allowances. (If a bereaved person often directs anger at you, see "Supporting others in grief: Suggestions for friends and family members," page 23.)

death is simply not possible or is of little importance. It can be expressed as numbness and disbelief. People often say plaintively, "I keep thinking this is a dream and I will wake up." When a death is unexpected, someone may insist, "But I saw him this morning and he was fine." But denial can take other forms, too, such as when someone brushes aside the importance or the impact of a death—saying, for example, "We never got along."

Denial can be troublesome when it suspends grieving. A person who is deeply mired in denial may find it hard to deal with harsh realities, such as the need to get treatment, admit that a parent is failing, plan a funeral, or pick up the pieces of a shattered life. But denial is not all bad. Sometimes the rush of painful truth is too tough to grapple with all at once. Little by little, as time goes by and a loss sinks in, people may move beyond denial to acceptance. That doesn't mean that denial disappears forever. Generally, it can still serve as a useful defense at times when unvarnished reality is too hard to bear.

For tips on dealing with denial, see "Managing denial," page 5.

Working through guilty feelings

Often people have unresolved issues in their relationships with their deceased loved ones. To feel whole again, it's important to work through any feelings of guilt you may have. These exercises may help.

Write a letter. Express your feelings to the person who died. Read it aloud in a favorite spot or perhaps in a place where you can feel his or her presence. Keep the letter with you so you can read it or add to it whenever you like. This may be especially helpful if you didn't get to say goodbye.

Consider good and bad. Write down the good things about the relationship or experiences you are glad to have shared. Then note what worked poorly in the relationship or things you wish you hadn't shared. Accept that people, including you, are imperfect. You can't always give or get love in the way you might wish to do so.

Talk to a friend. Try to find a good listener who won't attempt to tell you what you should be feeling. Discussing your true feelings with an empathetic friend, preferably one who's experienced a similar loss and can understand what you're going through, can help lighten the burden of guilt and may reveal other perspectives that you are overlooking (see "Turn to family and friends," page 15). Alternatively, confide in a minister, rabbi, priest, or grief counselor (see "Seek professional help," page 18).

For suggestions on handling angry feelings, see "Coping with anger," page 6.

Anger is common

People express anger in many ways and for many different reasons. It may appear as envy, bitterness, impatience, simmering resentment, explosive rage, or puzzlement over the unfairness of it all. Some people feel more comfortable getting angry than crying. Children who are grieving may express their feelings through frequent tantrums or irritability.

One problem with anger is that it often gets misdirected. Family, doctors, God, and entirely unrelated people or organizations may be the targets of intense anger, when the underlying emotion is anger about being abandoned by the person who died. Grieving people sometimes find that their anger bubbles over unexpectedly, pushing others away at times when their support could be helpful. Sometimes anger serves to hide other emotions—it's a secondary emotion masking the primary one.

The burden of guilt

Guilt evokes a sense of failure, remorse, and regret. Questions about what you might have done to avert the death may gnaw at you, and are a common and normal feature of grief, especially in the early phases. Or you may simply feel guilty if you were not present when your loved one died—a very common occurrence, since you cannot be by a dying person's bedside 24 hours a day, no matter how devoted you are. Guilt may also arise when a relationship was rocky and conflicts remain unresolved, or when the emotions you feel—numbness, anger, relief, or even surges of happiness—don't seem to jibe with what other people think you should feel. When a death follows a long or difficult illness, caregivers may feel guilty about feeling a sense of relief.

For some ideas on managing such emotions, see "Working through guilty feelings," above.

Making arrangements

After a loved one dies, you will find your life in the first several weeks taken over by the rituals of preparing a funeral or memorial service, making arrangements for a cremation or burial, writing an obituary, and taking care of paperwork such as death certificates.

Planning a meaningful funeral

Some people express their funeral wishes before they die, saying they want to have certain hymns at the service, for example, or be buried at sea, if they've served in the Navy or Marines. Be guided by what you know of your loved one's wishes. A funeral director or religious leader may be able to help you as well.

But note that while most people try to plan a funeral or memorial service that honors the wishes of the deceased—and there is something very satisfying about knowing that your loved one would have been pleased with the ceremony—ultimately these observances are for the comfort of the survivors. Plan a memorial that is meaningful to you and to those who mourn with you. Consider these questions:

- Do you want a traditional religious ceremony, or would you prefer to arrange a more personalized memorial in a place that held meaning to you both?
- Will a religious leader do all the talking, or do you want friends and family to share reminiscences? If so, who?
- Do you want to make any remarks yourself? If so, think about how your friend or family member approached life. Did he or she have a life philosophy you could relate? Is there a story that encapsulates this? What were his or her accomplishments and gifts—for example, volunteer or paid work, awards, great warmth, a knack for nurturing family ties, or a keen sense of humor? Think about what he or she was most proud of. What did you cherish most? What did you create or share together? Did your loved one have a favorite saying that you could relate to his or her life?
- What kind of music do you want? Did your loved one have any favorite songs or hymns? Do you?
- Are there passages that should be read from the Bible, the Koran, or any other religious or spiritual book?
- Is there meaningful poetry or inspirational or well-loved writings that could be read?
- Will you post favorite photographs of your loved one on a board near the entrance?
- When should you hold the funeral? Although some religions mandate a burial soon after death, many people need some time to collect themselves and begin to process the loss before a memorial service seems possible. Time may allow people to come from far away or prepare meaningful words.
- Do you want friends to come to the ceremony, or only close family members?
- Will guests come with you to the cemetery for the interment?
- Will there be a luncheon or reception afterward? If so, where?
- If your loved one was cremated, will you save some of the ashes to scatter later in your garden or a spot that meant a lot to you both?
- Should people send flowers? Or would a donation to a charity be a suitable, supportive gesture?

The planning form on page 9 will give you space to jot down some of your answers to these questions. Bear in mind that this is a time when even nontraditional or nonreligious relatives may want to observe traditional rituals. Culture and religion dictate certain customs. Rituals and routine also provide a sense of continuity and connection. Such practices can help you mark the loss and can feel comforting, particularly if you were raised with them. For example, if you are Greek, a traditional meal called a *makaria*, or "meal of mercy," might be served, and you may exchange greet-

Funeral or memorial service planning form

Did your loved one specify any wishes about burial, cremation, or body donation?

Who will handle the burial or cremation? Is there a pre-arranged plan or burial plot? If the body is to be donated to a medical school, is there an agreement in writing?

Who will pay the burial costs? Have any payments been made in advance? Is there burial insurance, or is the deceased entitled to veterans' benefits or other funds from the government, a union, or another organization to cover funeral costs?

What would you like to say on the tombstone?

Questions to consider when planning a service

When should the service be held?

Should the service be in a church, mosque, synagogue, or other religious gathering place? Have you contacted your religious leader? Or would you prefer an observance at your house, the funeral home, or the cemetery instead?

Are there family or cultural customs to follow?

What readings would you like at the ceremony?

Is there special music you would like to request?

Who should speak at the funeral or memorial?

Do you want to make any remarks yourself? Jot down ideas here.

Is there a special way for children to play a role?

Will you print a program listing readings, music, and speakers? Do you want it to include photographs?

Are there favorite pictures that could be displayed during the ceremony?

Do you want people to send flowers, or would you prefer that they contribute to a favorite charity? If so, which one, and what is the address?

Will any service be open to all, or only to family and possibly close friends? If the gathering is to be small, who should come?

Will there be a reception after the burial at someone's home or in another place? If so, what restaurant or caterer will you call?

Is there a family member or close friend who could help call people to tell them about the arrangements? Do you prefer to call people yourself?

What newspapers will you place obituaries in? What cities might your loved one still have contacts in, who would want to see the notice? Have you included information about the funeral plans, so that people you have not contacted might still get the word?

ings with family members, such as "May you have a full life" and "Memory is eternal." If you are from a Muslim tradition, your custom might be to spend the first few days of mourning socializing with family members, a practice aimed at easing grief. If you are Jewish, you might sit shiva, receiving visitors (who usually bring food and stories) at home for seven days after the death.

Once you know what you would like to do, spell out your wishes to friends and family members. People often make missteps because they are uncertain what you want. If you feel too exhausted and upset to talk about the subject, perhaps a family member or friend could help fill other people in. Keep in mind, though, that there are many different individual and cultural styles of grieving. Even if you communicate your wishes clearly, others may mourn the loss in a variety of ways.

There are also more prosaic details to think of, like finding a funeral home and figuring out how to pay the burial costs. Is there a prepaid burial plan? Does the deceased already own a burial plot? The planning form on page 9 can help you gather this information. Start by filling in the first few lines with as much information as you have, including instructions, directions, and phone numbers.

Covering costs

Just like the cost of living, the cost of dying—including the price of funerals and memorial services—is steadily rising. According to the National Funeral Directors Association, the average cost of a conventional funeral is around $7,200. And items many of us don't immediately consider—such as flowers, obituaries, and burial liners or vaults, among others—can push the price beyond $10,000.

At few times in life are people more vulnerable to sales pressure and blandishments than after the death of a loved one. Try not to let guilt or fear of what people will think guide your choices. Paying more than you can afford probably won't assuage pain, and it can certainly add to your worries. A simple, loving ceremony can dignify a person's memory as well as a lavish, costly one can.

Certain laws help protect people mourning a death. The Funeral Rule, enforced by the Federal Trade Commission (FTC), requires funeral homes to hand you written, itemized price lists of their services and detail them by phone, if asked. Such services might include consultation with the funeral director, a non-negotiable professional services and overhead fee, transportation and care of the body, use of the facilities for visitation and services, and other options. Casket prices must be detailed, too. Sometimes cremation costs are not completely spelled out if the crematory is off-premises, so ask about the full cost, including the cost of an urn or other container.

It's a good idea to contact several funeral homes. Differences in facilities, attitude, and cost may surprise you. The FTC offers a simple price checking sheet that can help you make comparisons, along with many helpful tips, in the publication "Shopping for Funeral Services," which can be downloaded from the agency's website at www.consumer.ftc.gov/articles/0070-shopping-funeral-services.

Under the federal Funeral Rule, funeral homes cannot charge extra if you choose to buy a casket from a different source. You can also choose individual services rather than buying a package. If you choose direct cremation or immediate burial, or if you donate the body to a medical school, you don't need to purchase a casket. (No embalming is done in these cases, and immediate burial requires only a simple container. There is no viewing or visitation, although you may elect to pay for a graveside service or memorial service.) Be aware that some cemeteries require burial

Avoiding funeral fraud

The Funeral Consumers Alliance is a nonprofit educational organization with member groups in many states. Its website (www.funerals.org) offers helpful advice about burial insurance plans, funeral service fees, caskets, cremation, choices for simple funerals, and many other topics. It also has tips on avoiding fraud and resolving complaints. Members may use cooperative buying power to reduce costs of caskets and funeral services.

The FTC offers a consumer guide to funeral planning. The FTC doesn't resolve individual complaints, but it may act against a company in some cases (see "Resources," page 44).

containers ("liners" or far more costly "vaults") that cover the casket and keep the ground from sinking unevenly. However, no health concerns require this, and some religions reject it.

One less costly option, "green" burial, is offered in a few parts of the country. Usually, a green burial means the body is not embalmed and is buried either without a casket or in a simple, biodegradable wooden one. A flat memorial rather than a gravestone may mark the grave.

In some cases, costs may be defrayed or covered entirely by prepaid burial plans, memorial societies, unions, professional organizations, the Department of Veterans Affairs, or the Social Security Administration. A funeral director may have other suggestions as well.

Gathering essential records

No matter how private a matter death is for you, it reverberates quite publicly. Within days and months of your loss, you'll need to gather many documents and make financial decisions. This may be less burdensome and confusing if you acquaint yourself with what you'll need and try to collect some of these items before you are pressed to do so.

Death, birth, and marriage certificates. The funeral director or county health department can issue death certificates. You may need several certified copies, since various agencies and companies will request this document before releasing information or funds. If you're applying for survivor's benefits, you'll also need birth and marriage certificates. Birth certificates are available through the public records department in the state or county where the person was born. Marriage certificates are filed with the county clerk where the marriage was performed. The National Center for Health Statistics website has state-by-state listings that can help you track down these vital documents and learn about fees for getting them (www.cdc.gov/nchs/nvss.htm).

A will. A copy of the will may be found grouped with other important papers, possibly in a safe deposit box. If a lawyer wrote it, he or she should have a copy.

Social Security numbers. You'll need the correct Social Security numbers for the deceased, spouse, and any children who are dependents. For help, you can contact the Social Security Administration at 800-772-1213 or go to the website at https://secure.ssa.gov.

Discharge papers for veterans. Next of kin can find request forms for discharge papers by going to www.archives.gov/veterans/military-service-records. You can also get a copy from the National Personnel Records Center at 1 Archives Drive, St. Louis, MO 63138 (call toll-free at 866-272-6272 or go to the site www.archives.gov/st-louis/military-personnel); the center is part of the National Archives.

Financial information. Make a list of property and important financial information. Include real estate and personal property, insurance policies and account numbers, stocks, bonds, deeds, leases, bank and credit union accounts, retirement accounts, pension fund information, and a federal income tax return from the previous year. If a copy of the tax return isn't available, file IRS form 4506 with the IRS to receive one. You can download this form from www.irs.gov.

Information about debts. Make a list of your loved one's regular bills and credit card accounts. If necessary, you can do so by going through past bills and checkbooks. Find out what outstanding debts he or she may have had, including a mortgage.

Contacting the appropriate agencies

You'll need to inform certain agencies and organizations about the death for financial and legal reasons. Most will require a certified death certificate, which you can obtain through the funeral home or the county health department in the county where the death occurred.

Insurance companies. If you are the beneficiary of your loved one's life insurance policy, you will want to notify the company as soon as possible to collect the funds. Find out if the deceased also made any arrangements to cover mortgages, other bank loans, and credit card debts. You also need to contact your loved one's health care insurer (whether a private insurer, Medicare, or Medicaid) as soon as possible to inform them of the death. If applicable, find out if your loved one had accident insurance or sudden death and dismemberment insurance.

U.S. Social Security Administration. If the deceased received Social Security benefits, contact this agency at www.ssa.gov or 800-772-1213 (toll-free) to report the death. If you're applying for survivor's benefits, you'll need to supply birth, marriage, and death certificates; Social Security numbers; and the last federal income tax return.

Other sources of funds and benefits. You may be eligible for certain burial or death benefits from other agencies, such as the Department of Veterans Affairs (VA) or the U.S. Office of Personnel Management. The VA defrays some funeral and burial costs; veterans and their spouses and dependent children can be buried at no cost in a national cemetery (so can some Public Health Service personnel); survivors may also receive educational or medical aid.

Employers. Your loved one may also have had life, accident, or health insurance coverage through a current employer or been owed for unused vacation or sick time. It's worth contacting his or her past employers, too, to ask if you're entitled to any death benefits. Also contact professional organizations and unions.

Banks. Banks can freeze funds in joint accounts in some states. If possible, before an anticipated death, ask your bank what laws govern joint accounts, and find out how funds can be released if an account is frozen. It may make sense to transfer money to a new account.

Creditors. Write or call all credit card companies and other creditors to explain the circumstances and cancel the accounts. Remember to copy all correspondence. If you speak with anyone on the phone, write down the person's name and extension number. Often, a certified death certificate (and occasionally other records) will be required in order to cancel the account. Also check bank and credit card accounts for automatic payments and renewals that may need to be canceled at death.

A probate lawyer. Probate is a public, legal process supervised by the courts after a person dies. It helps ensure that debts are paid and assets are properly owned and correctly distributed. Certain items do not go through probate, including jointly owned property (such as a house), property placed in a legal trust, and financial assets that have a designated beneficiary, such as life insurance policies and 401(k) accounts. If the deceased did not write a will, the estate will be divided among family members according to state law. A representative appointed by the court may oversee this. If there is a will, it will name an executor (also known as a personal representative in some states) to oversee the division of the estate.

You may need a lawyer to help guide you through the probate or trust process, especially if the estate was large or complicated. Find one who has experience with probate and estate issues. The AARP suggests asking what percentage of time the lawyer spends on probate cases. Also inquire about fees. If you're over 60, you may be able to get free legal assistance through your local agency or council on aging (check phone listings for a local agency). The American Bar Association and local bar associations sometimes offer free legal assistance to people in need. For simple estates, you probably don't need an attorney; ask a probate court clerk how to get information about the legal procedures required. Your public library and state or county bar association may be able to help, too.

Letting others know

These tasks are less urgent. But at some point, you will want to contact alumni magazines or newsletters of organizations your loved one was involved in. If your loved one maintained a holiday greeting card list of old friends you haven't seen for years, you'll want to let the people on this list know, too.

Coping with grief and loss

Losing someone close to you can be draining physically as well as emotionally. All the small details of daily life—getting out of bed, making meals, going to appointments, taking care of children, plowing through tasks tied to a household or work—may seem monumentally hard or inconsequential. Let the nonessentials slide, and focus on ways to help yourself through this difficult time.

Maintaining a healthy routine is important for everyone who's grieving a loss (see "Tend to the essentials," below). Beyond this, there is a lot you can do to comfort yourself. This chapter suggests many supportive strategies to try. But reading all of this at once or trying every suggestion at the same time would be overwhelming. Don't feel compelled to do that. Instead, dip into this chapter as needed. You may want to try focusing on just one suggestion at a time. Pick the ones that seem most likely to help you.

Tend to the essentials

When you are grieving, you may neglect yourself, but it's important to try to maintain your physical and mental well-being. Adequate sleep, nourishing food, and exercise can make you feel physically better, which in turn will improve your psychological outlook. Having a structure is helpful to most people.

Establish a simple, daily schedule. Getting back to a familiar routine after the death of a loved one can help restore a sense of normalcy and make grief more manageable. It lends structure to the day at a time when life seems unfamiliar and out of control. And it can help prevent you from falling into dangerous habits such as excessive alcohol use.

During the first few days after a loss, try to get out of bed at the same time, take a shower, and have breakfast. Create a "to-do" list for the day. While this might seem overwhelming at first, it can help you organize and prioritize your personal affairs. Include small things that give you comfort, such as a walk, a tasty bowl of soup, or a warm bath.

Maintain a regular sleep schedule. Even under normal circumstances, sleep is essential for optimal daily functioning—not just for alertness, but for physical health. Bereavement disrupts sleep cycles, which can contribute to difficulty coping and feeling overwhelmed. Poor sleep is also associated with elevated blood pressure, reduced immune function, and insulin resistance that can be a precursor of type 2 diabetes. But when you're grieving, sleep can be particularly important at helping maintain emotional balance. Grief is exhausting, and sleep can represent a relief from the emotional pain of loss.

Here are some ways to make sure you're getting the sleep you need:

- Use naps strategically. If possible, nap shortly after lunch. People who doze later in the afternoon tend to fall into a deeper sleep, which causes greater disruption to sleep at night. An ideal nap lasts no longer than an hour, and even a 15- to 20-minute nap has significant alertness benefits.
- Go to bed early if you can. If you're having trouble sleeping, try exercising more (but not in the evening).
- Avoid drinking beverages containing caffeine after 2 p.m., and abstain from alcohol for at least two hours before bedtime.

If these measures aren't sufficient, talk with your doctor. Sometimes, taking medication for a limited amount of time to help you sleep can help you cope better during the day. It's perfectly appropriate to take sleep medication in the weeks after losing a loved one.

Keep up with your exercise. When you are grieving, exercise may be the last thing you want to do, but it offers many benefits. Exercise can serve as a distraction when you need a break from grief, or offer you time to meditate on your loss. For a person who is grieving, exercise can also help lift spirits by releasing mood-elevating hormones, relieving stress, and promoting a sense of well-being. A simple walk, a bike ride, yoga, or a harder workout can ease agitation, anger, and depression. In some studies, exercising regularly eased mild to moderate depression as effectively as medications.

Eat well. Many people who are grieving find that they lose their appetite; others find themselves eating more than usual, or less healthily than usual. Consuming nourishing food will help your body function as well as possible during this stressful time. Avoid foods that supply mostly empty calories, like candy, chips, cookies, and pastries. Drink plenty of fluids, and limit alcohol and caffeinated drinks. If you've lost your appetite, try simple comfort foods, such as soups, mashed potatoes with chicken or meatloaf, fruit and yogurt smoothies, puddings, pasta, or foods from your childhood or cultural background. Eating small portions frequently may help, too. Take a multivitamin to cover any nutrients your diet isn't currently supplying.

Take necessary medications. Grief makes you more vulnerable to illness. Keep taking your regular medicines. Not everyone needs an antidepressant or anti-anxiety medication, but these drugs can be lifesaving for some people. Talk with your doctor about this, if necessary.

Stop (or don't start) risky behavior. It is very tempting, when you are grieving, to want a glass of wine or scotch to relax; if you find yourself drinking more than usual, if others around you are worried about your drinking, or if you feel like your drinking is getting more difficult to control, these are danger signs that suggest that limiting your intake is essential. Other dangerous coping strategies include abusing drugs or engaging in impulsive or risky behavior. These may blot out or numb pain temporarily, but they ultimately derail healthy grieving and can have other unwanted consequences. Substituting safer behaviors when these impulses arise—such as seeking solace with other caring people, praying, exercising, writing in a journal, or trying stress-relief techniques—will serve you better. If you are finding yourself drawn to risky behaviors, you may want to contact a grief counselor or mental health professional who can help you make healthier choices as you grieve (see "What is a grief counselor?" on page 19).

Delay big decisions. In the throes of grief, many people consider making big changes—moving, changing jobs, throwing out keepsakes, and so forth. Grief can cloud your thought processes, and if you make abrupt decisions, you may regret them later. Many experts suggest waiting a year, if possible, before making momentous decisions.

See your doctor. After a loss, any upsetting physical symptoms may be magnified and can make you feel terribly alone. It's not unusual to have symptoms similar to those of the person who died. A visit to your doctor can identify ailments that could put you further under the weather, or may just restore peace of mind. Keep up with routine health care, too, such as regular physical exams and dental appointments and any medical tests you need.

Give yourself permission to grieve. Grief is painful, and there is a strong drive to "finish" grieving quickly, to relieve your misery. But you need to know that healing won't happen immediately. Be patient with yourself. Bear in mind that many tasks take longer when you are grieving. Ask, "What would help me most today?" The answer may vary from day to day and even from hour to hour. If you need to cry, cry. If you feel angry, express it. If you feel guilty, explore it. If you need support from friends or family—a hug, a home-cooked dinner, a night out, or just their presence in your home—tell someone. If you need a break from grieving, allow yourself that. If you're afraid of the feelings you're having, share them with a caring friend or family member, a support group of people treading the same path, a religious leader, a spiritual counselor, or a mental health professional. Holidays can be particularly difficult (see "Handling holidays and difficult times," page 15).

Do something for yourself every day. There are many tasks to take care of in the aftermath of a death, from writing the obituary, obtaining death certificates, and arranging the memorial service or funeral in the near term to longer-term tasks like dealing with the estate and probate. In the midst of it all, be sure you make time for yourself, too. Small pleasures can help remind you of the joy that is still possible in your life.

Handling holidays and difficult times

Holidays, anniversaries, birthdays, and events that would otherwise be joyful can be especially hard on people who are grieving. If your grief is fresh, holiday cheer can seem like an affront. Celebrations may underscore how alone you feel. Likewise, it's hard to accept that others may not mark the days that you do—the first time you met, a birthday, or the anniversary of an illness or death. The following strategies may help ease your pain around holidays and other difficult times.

Be with people. Even though you may not feel like it, social contact is usually comforting. Choose people you feel comfortable with. Share what is on your mind. Remind them that they don't need to "fix" your pain, but that it would be helpful for them to listen.

Start a new tradition or build on an old one. Remember the deceased on special occasions by placing a lighted candle on the table, leaving an empty chair, or saying a few words of remembrance. If the person who died always played a special role in festivities, ask another family member to carry on the tradition.

Ask for advice. Talk to others who have lost people close to them to find out how they have managed holidays.

Change the celebration. Opt for a simpler celebration. Go out to dinner instead of planning an elaborate meal at home. Schedule a trip or an outing with family members or friends.

Express your needs. Let others know that you may not participate in all the festivities this year or that you need to let go of overwhelming or unsatisfying traditions. Feel free to tell people you're just not up to it right now or to change plans at the last minute. Don't feel pressured to do more than you want to do. Cry if you need to. Leave an event when you wish to.

Plan to mark the day. Walk through a nature preserve. Visit the cemetery or the place where ashes were scattered. Enjoy an activity the deceased would also have loved, tell a joke she would have appreciated, or perform a service for others in his honor. Think of a ritual to help you connect. Light a candle and say a prayer. Release balloons. Carry a memento from your loved one. Meditate. Tell someone you're close to how you feel and why. Ask people to share their memories of the deceased with you.

Help someone else. Volunteer to help others through a charitable or religious organization. Make a donation to a favorite cause in memory of the person who died.

Planning for the first anniversary of a death

It's not just birthdays, holidays, and other cheerful occasions that are tough. The first anniversary of your loved one's death is a particularly significant day. Anticipate that it's likely to be a challenging time. Plan to be with people you're close to. Maybe you want to host a dinner and have everyone tell stories about your loved one. Maybe you and your children want to visit the gravesite or a place that was special to all of you. Or perhaps you want to bring out some old letters and photographs to look at. Sharing these things will likely ease your loneliness.

Maybe you treat yourself to a cappuccino or go to dinner with a friend—whatever qualifies as "you" time. Sue Morris, a grief counselor at the Dana-Farber Cancer Institute in Boston and the author of *Overcoming Grief: A Self-Help Guide Using Cognitive Behavioral Techniques*, goes one step further and calls for creating your own "grief spa." Like a conventional spa, where you go to pamper and care for yourself, a grief spa should serve as a source of comfort and renewal. The "spa menu" will vary according to your personal preferences. The self-care toolkit in one person's spa, for example, might include writing in a journal, doing yoga, attending a bereavement group, volunteering in the community, and getting a pet. Another's might consist of listening to music, getting regular massages, creating a memory book, being with friends, and joining an online support group. New activities can be added and old ones eliminated as needs change and emerge. What's important is for you to find things that help your outlook.

Keep track of "small wins." Every day, try writing down three things that have gone well. At a later stage, you might try keeping a gratitude journal that records fleeting things that actually made you feel good (see "Keep a journal," page 20). But at this early stage, just write down small victories like managing to go to the gym or eating a healthy meal. Over time, this can help you rebuild a sense of normalcy.

Turn to family and friends

If you are fortunate, family and friends can provide a strong source of support. Often, a death prompts people to think about what's important in life. It can break down barriers built up years ago and motivate people to help one another. The compassionate gestures of friends and family cannot be underestimated in times of grief and bereavement. Whether these gestures are small or large, the kindness of loved ones can sustain and console you in a difficult time.

While some may surround you with love, others may actively take a step back from you. A few may be full of unhelpful, even hurtful, comments. Alan D. Wolfelt, a grief counselor and author of *Healing Your Grieving Heart* and *Healing the Adult Child's Grieving Heart*, suggests identifying three people who can staunchly support you in the coming weeks and months. Think about who is the most helpful and the least judgmental in your circle. Ask them whether they can help by listening to you when you need to talk and spending time with you when you need support.

Of course, there are times and situations when such encouragement is not readily available. In these circumstances, a counselor or bereavement group can provide needed support.

The following tips may also be useful.

Tell people what helps. You might say, "I just need to cry right now," or "There's nothing you can do to fix this. It helps if you just stay with me." If you want to talk about the person you're missing, let others know. For example, say, "I just want to talk about her, but I feel like everyone is afraid to say her name."

Be honest about your feelings. Feelings differ from person to person, but if you're not sure how to begin the conversation, these examples may help:

- "I feel so angry about Mike's death. It seems so useless."
- "I'm relieved that Mom isn't suffering anymore, but I miss her terribly."
- "My relationship with my dad was really difficult. I'm feeling a lot of things right now—not just sadness."
- "I know you think I should be over this, but I'm not."

Take away uncertainty. Often, people aren't sure how to act around you. Should they mention your loved one's name, or will that make you sadder? Should they reach out and hug you? Should they offer advice? Are you angry with them? Is it all right to share a joke or a funny memory? Doing so yourself can encourage others to do the same. In general, it will help if you can provide clear signals. For example, you might say things like these:

- "I'm finding it really hard to get out of the house. Could we make a regular date to walk or have dinner or maybe see a movie?"

Religion and spirituality

Religion and spirituality are, for many, the beacons of light that offer guidance and comfort on bereavement's dark journey. For these people, spiritual or religious rituals are a great consolation. Whether this means sitting shiva, setting up an altar inside the home, or gathering at the cemetery once a year, such rituals can draw people together and encourage them to express their grief.

Drawing on other aspects of your religious or spiritual life can help as well. If prayer heartens or sustains you, set aside time for it. Read spiritual texts that you find comforting, attend services, and share your circumstances with a religious leader who can help place the death in the context of your faith.

On a very practical level, attending religious services can link you with a well-defined community primed to offer help of all sorts: a kind word, a willing listener, a shared meal, or any one of a number of large and small acts of assistance help keep you afloat and ease your distress after a death. Whatever form of belief—or nonbelief—an ill person or grieving loved one embraces, illness and loss inevitably set in motion an examination of meaning and the fleeting nature of life. Identifying people with whom you can share these questions and the feelings they bring up represents an opportunity for growth and healing.

On another level, religious or spiritual beliefs may lend larger meaning to a loved one's life and death. Each life is significant, whether long or short, and, in the view of most religions, equally cherished. Seeing your loved one's life as part of a grander plan may help. Religion often presents a view, too, on how the deceased fares after death. Surely it could help ease a sore heart to believe that a loved one is enjoying the spiritual riches of heaven or preparing for the next turn of the wheel through reincarnation. Believing your loved one helps guide you in this world or that you will be reunited in another place after your own death can bring comfort, help you continue to feel connected with the person, and make you feel less alone.

- “If you really want to help, cleaning up the kitchen or vacuuming would be great.”
- “I can’t bear to be alone tonight, but I don’t want to talk. Could you stay and just watch TV with me?”
- “Sometimes I make plans and find later that I’m just not up to following through with them. I hope you’ll understand if that happens.”
- “I feel so mad about everything, I’m snapping at everyone all the time.”
- “Hugs just make me feel worse right now. What I need is a little time alone.”

Spend time with others who understand. If others in your family or among your friends have also lost a loved one, they may be more empathetic. You can ask outright: “What helped you? How did you get through this awful time?” They may recall having the same feelings you’re finding so alarming now—whether it’s numbness and no tears, waves of guilt, fury, confusion and anxiety, or a seemingly bottomless well of sorrow. When friends and family can’t help in these ways, support groups often can (see “Join a grief support group,” below right).

Reach out to your religious community, if applicable. Even those who have fallen away from their faith over the years may find comfort in reconnecting with the traditions of their youth (see “Religion and spirituality,” page 16).

Leave the door open. You may wish everyone would just go away and leave you alone to sort through your feelings. If you express yourself too forcefully, though, you may drive people further away than you mean to at a time when you truly need their support. Try to leave the door open a bit. Here are some things you might say:

- “I just want to go home and go to bed right now. Would you call me tomorrow, though?”
- “I feel so upset these days, I can’t settle on anything. Please don’t take it personally.”
- “I’m just not up to that right now. Maybe in a few weeks. Will you try me again?”

Realize that different people grieve differently. You may not be the only mourner. Others may be grieving the same loss in their own ways. For example, two parents grieving a child’s loss may react differently. One might need to cry and talk frequently.

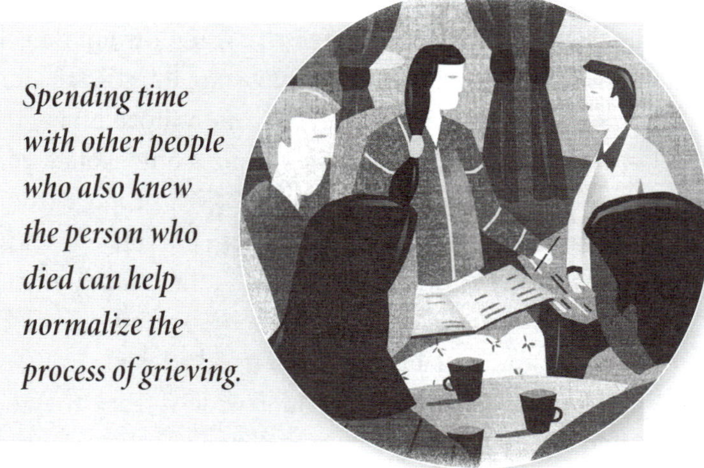

Spending time with other people who also knew the person who died can help normalize the process of grieving.

The other might work incessantly and act increasingly distant. Both are trying desperately to deal with their pain and loss. Professional insight from a grief counselor can be valuable when grieving drives a wedge between you and your partner, family members, or others who are important to you (see “What is a grief counselor?” on page 19).

Understand that personal items may hold special meaning for others. After a significant loss, it’s not uncommon for the deceased’s personal items, large and small, to take on special meaning. Sometimes family members find themselves squabbling over clothes, jewelry, furniture, or other belongings. Accusations of greed or coldness may fly, for example, as one adult child seeks many belongings, while another suggests ways to dispose of as much as possible as quickly as possible. If this occurs, think and talk about the emotional reasons behind the dispute for all parties. Try to remember that people may have very strong feelings about possessions because of what they represent and the memories that they hold.

Join a grief support group

A sounding board, a voice of experience, people to share with—a good grief support group promises many things. Should you join one? That depends on your circumstances. Don’t feel pressured to do so. But if you think you could benefit from talking about your experiences and hearing about those of others, you may find a group quite helpful.

Sometimes friends and family members shy away from strong emotions and sad topics. You may feel they just don't understand what you're going through. Even caring friends and relatives may start to indicate subtly or outright that it's time for you to move on before you're ready to do so. These attitudes only isolate you further and make you feel worse. A grief support group can offer understanding and a sense of connection. In the company of others treading a similar path, you can express strong feelings, validate the varied emotions you feel, and possibly even hear good advice.

Grief support groups differ widely. They may be open to anyone or focus on particular diseases or situations, such as a group for widowers or bereaved children. Some groups are ongoing; others convene for a specific length of time. Groups may charge fees, which are sometimes covered by health insurance. Certain organizations consist of a network of self-help groups. Through the group Compassionate Friends, for example, parents who have experienced grief after the death of a child of any age reach out to other parents in similar circumstances.

A local hospice, hospital, or community organization may be able to guide you to a group that is capably led and seems to be a good fit. Your doctor, a therapist, or a religious organization might also be able to help you locate a support group.

If a group feels uncomfortable or you're unsure if it's the right fit, try talking to the group facilitator. After trying a few sessions, if you find that focusing on your grief makes you feel worse or you don't think the group is right for you, then don't feel compelled to stick around. In that case, you might consider one-on-one counseling.

What makes grieving harder?

Getting through grief is always difficult, but research shows certain factors can make it harder. The path tends to be rougher if you

- had a highly dependent relationship with the deceased
- have experienced multiple deaths or important losses
- have suffered from depression or another mental illness
- have low self-esteem.

Circumstances surrounding the death also make a difference. Grieving may be harder if

- the death was unexpected or untimely
- the death was traumatic or violent
- the death was from suicide, a stigmatized illness such as AIDS, or a drug overdose
- you bear some responsibility for the death, such as involvement in a car or gun accident
- you helped care for the deceased for more than six months
- you were unable to perform cultural rituals of importance to you
- you have little social support
- you have few opportunities to meet others or engage in new pursuits
- you are under stress from other crises.

If any of these apply, consider whether you may need extra time or support to deal with your grief. Joining a grief support group or talking with a spiritual or grief counselor or therapist might be especially helpful in these circumstances.

Seek professional help

While it's not necessary for everyone who is grieving to seek professional assistance, working with a counselor or therapist who specializes in grief may be helpful for some. Perhaps you feel that you need assistance in coping with your sorrow but don't think a support group is right for you. Or maybe you're finding that time hasn't eased your grief. Perhaps you suspect that you are struggling with depression or complicated grief (see "Depression and complicated grief," page 3, and "What makes grieving harder?" at left).

In such cases, you may find it helpful to turn to a mental health professional. It may also be useful if you are dealing with issues that are too complex or far-reaching to discuss in a support group—for example, if you had a very conflicted relationship with the person who died or you are coping with a traumatic death. Working one-on-one with a grief counselor or social worker, psychologist, or psychiatrist may make it easier for you to share your feelings and focus on your needs (see "What is a grief counselor?" on page 19). A psychiatrist can also help evaluate whether you might benefit from medication, such as an antidepressant or an anti-anxiety drug.

Another type of therapy that may help is cognitive behavioral therapy. Therapists can help you realize that many of the unhelpful ideas that are causing you anguish ("I will never be happy again," "My life is over") are not actually true. The therapist can help you start reframing your thoughts in more positive, less catastrophic ways.

Start your search for a good mental health professional by gathering referrals for a grief specialist from your doctor and people you trust. Once you have a few names, call to learn more about the following aspects of treatment:

Qualifications. Ask the counselor or therapist to describe his or her training. A grief therapist should be trained and licensed as a psychiatrist, psychologist, or social worker.

Experience. Ask how much experience the counselor or therapist has with the issues you are facing. How much of his or her practice is devoted to this? How much is devoted to people in the same age range? This is especially important when asking on behalf of bereaved children and teens.

Goals. Ask what the goals are for counseling or therapy. Goals differ depending on needs, of course. One goal might be to help you explore and resolve issues that may be interfering with healthy grieving, such as an idealized image of the person who died, angry or conflicted feelings about the deceased, or the weight of multiple losses or earlier losses that were never fully mourned. Others could be to encourage healthy expressions of grief and guide you toward adopting helpful coping strategies.

Cost. Discuss fees and health insurance coverage issues. Also ask about the number of sessions covered under your plan.

Fit. It's important that you feel comfortable with the therapist. An initial meeting can help you decide if this is a good fit. A good fit depends partly on a professional's personality and approach, as well as experience.

What is a grief counselor?

Grief counselors are specialists who are trained in grief counseling, a form of psychotherapy that helps individuals process and make sense of their feelings of loss and mourning. A key part of grief counseling is validation. Individuals who are grieving need to know that the signs and symptoms of grief that they are experiencing are normal.

Grief counselors also help people to understand that there are many ways to express and come to terms with grief. They are particularly attuned to common reactions to grief, whether these reactions are physical, emotional, or cognitive.

Check out books

Sometimes grief can make you feel terribly alone. No one seems to grasp what you're going through. The fog won't lift. Sleep is irregular, your appetite is gone, and your mind seems to have slowed. At any moment, your emotions may seem crushing or perversely out of whack with what you think you ought to feel. Newfound fears and erratic moods may prompt you to wonder about your mental health.

At such moments, good books and recordings on bereavement provide a safe, nonjudgmental haven. They spell out typical courses of grief and present coping strategies for you to try. Stories shared by others who have gone through this before you can be comforting and inspiring. You can pick up a book when you feel the urge and drop it again when you don't.

If friends or family members have been bereaved, ask them to suggest books they found helpful. Some examples appear in the "Resources" section of this report (page 44). Other good sources of suggestions are organizations that help the bereaved, hospice or grief counselors, and support groups.

Commemorate your loved one

Aside from the funeral, wake, or memorial service, you may find it helpful to commemorate the person in other ways. Remembering and honoring the person who died helps you keep memories alive. Sometimes it helps shape meaning from loss. If you would like to do this but aren't sure where to start, the suggestions that follow may be helpful.

A scrapbook. Create an album memorializing your loved one's life. Or try making a timeline of important dates and doings. Paste pictures in the scrapbook and write down stories, remembered sayings, and well-loved recipes. You might invite friends and family to write down stories, thoughts, or what they loved best about the person who died, especially if people are gathering for a memorial service or funeral. You may also want to share these stories with friends and family.

An online memorial. One example is a Facebook page in your loved one's memory. Encourage friends and family to add photos and reminiscences. You may be surprised at some of the stories you've never heard or photos you've never seen before. And you may be impressed at the number of people who want to contribute. Such a page can help you find community at a time when you might otherwise be isolated.

A memory box. Pictures, objects, and art supplies can be brought together to make a memory box for display or keepsakes. When you're ready to go through belongings, set aside items for a memory box.

A slide show. Favorite pictures and songs or sayings can be melded into a poignant multimedia remembrance of a life. Download photos into a digital picture frame. Old videos can also be revived and spliced together, then copied on DVDs for others to enjoy. Your local video or photo shop or a technology-minded friend or family member may be able to help with these projects.

A photo wall. Create a remembrance wall or collage of photos taken at different times and events.

Artwork. You might use art to explore your feelings, chronicle the life of the person who died, or express your ideas of an afterlife, if any. Children struggling with grief may find creating art—whether it's with clay, colored pens, paints, or collage supplies—particularly helpful. A memory quilt incorporating meaningful scenes and fabrics may be comforting.

A good cause. Violence prevention, medical research, peace efforts, scholarship funds, and many other causes have been taken up to honor someone's memory. Think about how the person you love would want to be remembered in the world. Reach out to a nonprofit organization devoted to helping prevent others' suffering. For example, a woman whose son is killed in a car crash caused by a drunk driver might channel her hurt and rage by developing presentations for high school students on the dangers of drunk driving. In this way, she transforms her feelings into a positive force that helps others.

A peaceful spot. Create a peaceful nook with a comfortable chair, lighting, photos, inspirational books, or other important objects in honor of your loved one. Build a serene spot with a fountain outside in your garden. Walk regularly through a nature preserve, or visit a spot your friend or family member particularly enjoyed.

A garden. Planting a garden or a tree can be a wonderful way to remember someone. You might want to offer flowers from the garden to others for their enjoyment or put them in an arrangement that you can bring to the cemetery. If the tree is not at your home, visiting it every year on your loved one's birthday can become a comforting ritual.

The gravesite. In many cultures, the gravesite is a focal point for commemorating the loved one, particularly on special days such as birthdays, anniversaries, or holy days. Plant flowers. Say a prayer, or simply visit for a few moments of contemplation.

A prayer. Spirituality is of great comfort to many people. Say prayers, light incense or a candle, create a shrine, ring bells, or participate in any spiritual activity that is meaningful to you.

An echo. Do something silly, pleasurable, or solemn that the deceased once did. Give a holiday toast, travel, take friends to a comedy, play well-loved music, crack a bad joke, or commit acts of kindness he or she would have appreciated.

Keep a journal

Some people hate writing, in which case keeping a journal may be no help at all. But others will want to remember the details of what they've experienced—details that can quickly disappear into the confusion and memory fog of grief. Keeping a journal can provide a valuable record, and can also help you sort through the rush of emotions you're experiencing at this time. If you wish to try journal writing, here are some guidelines to keep in mind:

- Truly let go. Write down what you feel and why you

feel that way. You're writing for yourself, not others. Don't worry about grammar or sentence structure.

- You may cry or feel deeply upset when writing. Nonetheless, many people find journal writing valuable and report feeling relief afterward.
- Try writing for 15 to 30 minutes a day for three to four days, or as long as a week if you feel writing continues to be helpful. Alternatively, try writing for 15 to 30 minutes once a week for a month. An analysis of multiple studies on journal writing, published in the *Journal of Consulting and Clinical Psychology*, showed that writing is more helpful when it extends over more days, and has the potential to improve your physical health, psychological well-being, and general functioning.

Some people also advocate keeping a gratitude journal. Although it may seem difficult at first to feel grateful for anything, you may find that after the initial shock of loss has worn off, it helps to write down something every day that brought a fleeting smile to your face. Maybe you heard a joke on TV that gave you a brief moment of pleasure or you received a kind word from a friend. Maybe a friend invited you over for dinner and you enjoyed trading stories about your loved one. Realize that even in the midst of this deep sorrow, you can feel moments of pleasure—and know that these moments will multiply as time moves on.

Note that deeply troubling situations, such as suicide or a violent death, are best explored with an experienced therapist. A therapist can help you to examine any unresolved issues you may have had with your loved one; treat you for post-traumatic stress disorder, if appropriate; and aid you in coping with the reactions of other family members.

De-stress with relaxation techniques

Stress can skyrocket during bereavement. The massive adjustments demanded of you can repeatedly trigger the stress response, a cascade of hormones that prepares your body to fight a foe or flee from imminent danger. Unless feelings of stress are given an outlet, physical and psychological symptoms—such as a clenched jaw, shakiness, and anxious feelings—tend to compound. This fuels a negative, self-perpetuating cycle of stress.

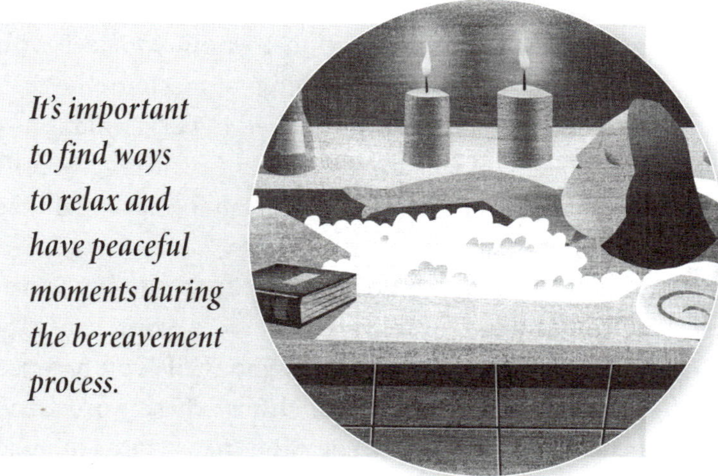
It's important to find ways to relax and have peaceful moments during the bereavement process.

Bereavement stirs up many sources of stress. Tempers may flare among family members brought together by a death. Finances may be pinched. Work obligations may loom within days of the funeral. The gap between all that needs to be done and all you feel you can do may widen every day. No wonder researchers have noted heightened levels of key stress hormones in bereaved subjects. Many investigators believe that over time these physiological changes trigger physical ailments. They may even help explain higher rates of death among certain groups, such as elderly widowers.

Research shows that health problems occur when the body repeatedly launches the stress response or never fully switches it off following a traumatic event. Consistently high blood pressure, which plays a central role in heart disease, has been linked to long-term stress. The buildup of stress often feeds or causes depression and anxiety, too.

One well-established way to counter stress is to invoke what's known as the "relaxation response"—for instance, with various forms of meditation. However, many people are too distracted to meditate, even when they're not coping with the effects of such a loss. If this sounds familiar, you may want to try a simpler technique called breath focus. Here's how:

1. Find a comfortable, quiet place to sit. When you are comfortably seated, place one hand on your lower belly. First try taking a normal breath. Now try a slow, deep breath. The air coming in through your nose should move downward, expanding your lungs fully so that your lower belly expands. Alternate between normal and deep breathing several times, paying attention to how you feel with each breath. Shallow breathing—especially the fast, panicky shallow breathing called hyperventilation—can make you feel anxious. Deep breathing, by contrast, slows your heart rate and can lower or stabilize blood pressure.

2. Breathe to a count, or choose a focus word. A focus word or phrase enhances your sense of peace, relaxation, and connection while you practice breath focus or other meditations. These words may be secular or religious; common focus words include "Peace" or "Om." They can have deep personal meaning or simply be pleasing. Repeat these words mentally as you perform the exercise. You might say one word or phrase to yourself as you breathe in and another as you breathe out, or just use one word or phrase as you exhale. Alternatively, you can breathe to a count—say, breathing in to a count of four and out to a count of eight. Long, slow exhaling is particularly relaxing.

3. Bring these elements together. As you sit comfortably with your eyes closed, blend deep breathing with a count or a focus word or phrase. Imagine that the air you breathe in washes peace and calm into your body. As you breathe out, imagine that the air leaving your body carries tension and sadness with it. Disregard distracting thoughts. Any time your attention drifts, simply say "Oh, well" to yourself and return to your breathing and counting or silent repetition of your focus word or phrase.

Try to practice breath focus for 10 to 20 minutes daily, preferably at the same time of day. If that goal seems impossible, try it for a few minutes whenever you feel symptoms of stress.

Mini-relaxation exercises

Mini-relaxations can be practiced almost anytime and anywhere. They are especially helpful when you feel signs of stress building up.

Letting pain recede

When grief is new, the pain feels fresh and sharp. As time goes on, it often dulls or recedes entirely for long stretches. That can seem oddly sad—as if holding on to pain is a measure of respect or duty and letting go means betraying someone you love or forever breaking ties that bind you. Try not to equate clinging to pain with holding on to the person who died. A strong connection can be maintained in other ways.

When you have one minute. Place your hand just beneath your navel so you can feel the gentle rise and fall of your belly as you breathe. Breathe in deeply, pause for a count of three, exhale, and then pause for a count of three. Continue to breathe deeply for one minute, pausing for a count of three after each inhalation and exhalation.

When you have three minutes. While seated, take a break to check your body for tension. Relax your facial muscles and allow your jaw to fall open slightly. Let your shoulders drop. Let your arms fall to your sides. Allow your hands to loosen so that there are spaces between your fingers. Uncross your legs or ankles. Feel your thighs sink into your chair, letting your legs fall comfortably apart. Feel your shins and calves become heavier and your feet grow roots into the floor. Now breathe in slowly. Breathe out slowly. Each time you exhale, try to relax even more.

When you have 10 minutes or more. Try visualization. Start by sitting comfortably in a quiet room. Bring your awareness to your breath for a few minutes. Now picture yourself in a place that conjures up good memories. What do you smell—the heavy scent of roses on a hot day, crisp fall air, the wholesome smell of baking bread? What do you hear? Drink in the colors and shapes that surround you. Focus on sensory pleasures: the swoosh of a gentle wind; soft, cool grass tickling your feet; the salty smell and rhythmic beat of the ocean.

Supporting others in grief: Suggestions for friends and family members

It can be hard to know how to console a friend or relative who is grieving. If it seems that nothing you can do or say helps, don't give up. You can't take the pain away, but your presence is more important than it seems. Accept that you can't fix the situation or make your friend or relative feel better. Instead just be present and offer hope and a positive outlook toward the future. Recognize that grieving is a gradual process.

Even small gestures—sending a card or flowers, delivering a meal, helping out with laundry or shopping, or making a regular date to listen and offer support—can be a huge source of comfort to a person who is grieving. One woman, a dog lover who had recently lost her husband, recalled her joy when a close friend went to the pound and brought her a basket of puppies that needed to be fostered for a few weeks.

It's important to be flexible and open to a person's way of grieving. For example, if a bereaved friend or family member is coming to your house for the holidays, ask if you can do anything to help mark the loss during this occasion. Be willing to leave plans loose. Build in a loophole when you extend the invitation: "We would love to have you join us. You needn't decide until the last minute, if you want some time to think about it." Gently press a person to accept your invitation, but take "no" for an answer without ire. Call the next day to check in.

It is sometimes difficult to know what to say to a bereaved person. If you find yourself tongue-tied or uncertain of what to do in the face of someone's loss, here are some ideas to help you.

Name names. Don't be afraid to mention the deceased. It won't make your friend any sadder, although it may prompt tears. It's terrible to feel that someone you love must forever be expunged from memory and conversation. Saying how much you'll miss the person is much better than the perfunctory, "I'm sorry for your loss."

Don't ask, "How are you?" The answer is obvious—"not good"—and because it's the same greeting you would offer anyone, it doesn't acknowledge that your friend has suffered a devastating loss. Instead try, "How are you feeling today?"

Offer hope. People who have gone through grieving often remember that it is the person who offered reassuring hope, the certainty that things will get better, who helped them make the gradual passage from pain to a renewed sense of life. Be careful, though, about being too glib, as doing so may make the bereaved person feel even more isolated. Rather, say something like: "You will grieve for as long as you need to, but you are a strong person, and will find your way through this." This remark both acknowledges that there is no quick and easy solution and also affirms your confidence that things will improve.

Reach out. Call to express your sympathy. Try to steer clear of such phrases as "It's God's will" or "It's for the best" unless the bereaved person says this first. Your friend or relative may need you even more after the first few weeks and months, when other people may stop calling. Check in every now and then just to say hello (you may find it helpful to put reminders on your calendar). Most bereaved people find it difficult to reach out and need others to take the initiative.

Practice your listening skills and ask general questions such as "How are you feeling today?" when visiting with a grieving person.

Help out. Don't just ask if you can "do anything." That transfers the burden to the bereaved, and he or she may be reluctant to make a request. Instead, be specific when offering help. Bring dinner over, pass on information about funeral arrangements, or answer the phone. Pitch in to clean up the kitchen. Sometimes your help is most valuable later. A lawyer might help answer questions about the estate. A handy person might button up the house as winter approaches.

Assist with meals. Provide hands-on assistance with cooking, and volunteer to help with shopping. For many bereaved persons, particularly widows and widowers, it can be a big adjustment to get accustomed to planning meals, shopping for groceries, and cooking for just one person.

Do the driving. Relatives in town for the funeral or memorial service may need a lift. Volunteer to ferry people to the funeral or to take children to activities on certain days. Grief can hamper driving abilities, so offer to drive your friend to appointments, too.

Write a note. If you had a relationship with the deceased, try to include a warm, caring, or funny anecdote that shows how wonderfully special he or she was. If you didn't know the deceased, offer your sympathy and assure the bereaved that he or she is in your thoughts or prayers. It is never too late to send a condolence note. A late note can provide comfort and offer an opportunity to remember the deceased in a new light.

Be sensitive to differences. People mourn and grieve in different ways. Religion plays a big role in how death is treated; so do ethnic, cultural, and family backgrounds. Avoid criticizing the funeral arrangements or memorial service. Also, try not to impose your beliefs about death on your friend.

Make a date. Ask your friend to join you for a walk or meal once a week. Be aware that weekends are often very difficult, and suggest an activity then. Low-stress activities may be best: watch a video at home together versus going out to a movie. Sometimes just being there without saying much is enough—it may even be exactly what your friend wants. If you're not sure what's wanted, offer several different options. Say something like: "I am cooking a big pot of soup tonight. Would you come over and join us?" Don't take it personally if your friend rebuffs offers or doesn't return every phone call. Keep trying.

Listen well instead of advising. A sympathetic ear is a wonderful thing. A friend who listens even when the same story is told with little variation is even better. Often, people work through grief and trauma by telling their story over and over. Unless you are asked for your advice, don't be quick to offer it. Frequently, those who are grieving really wish others would just listen. It's your understanding—not your advice—that is most sorely needed.

Avoid judgments. Your friend's life and emotional landscape have changed enormously, possibly forever. You may wish he or she would move on, but you can't speed the process or even ensure that it happens. Let your friend heal at the pace that feels right and in his or her own manner. "You should cry" or "It's time to move on" aren't really helpful directions.

Acknowledge difficult days. Some people appreciate hearing that you're thinking of them at difficult times, such as holidays, birthdays, and anniversaries. Take your cues from your friend, however. Sad reminders may make some feel worse.

Express your feelings. If you share your friend's sorrow, say so. It's even all right to blurt out that you don't know what to say. Most likely, nothing you say will turn the tide, but your sympathetic presence may make your friend feel slightly less alone. If you're concerned that your friend is slipping into a major depression or isn't feeling any better a year later, suggest that he or she talk with a mental health professional.

Handle anger gently. People who are grieving sometimes direct angry feelings toward the closest target. If that happens to be you, try to be understanding. Wait until well after the person has cooled down before raising your concern in a nonthreatening way. Being condescending or critical isn't helpful. So, rather than saying, "I think you owe me an apology," it may help to observe, "You seem angry a lot lately. I've been wondering if you're mad at me for something."

Keep your promises. If you offer to do anything, follow through. This is especially important where promises to children are involved. For a child, losing a loved one is abandonment enough.

Life stages and losses

Bereavement affects people differently at different stages in life. This is especially true of children, who are often the forgotten mourners. Grief in midlife and later years can vary, too. And whether the person you're mourning is your child, parent, sibling, or spouse also makes a difference.

Grief in the later years

Although people experience losses at every age, the toll mounts as one grows older. As friends and relatives pass away, the possibility arises of grief overload, which can lead to emotional numbness, depression, or complicated grief. This is particularly common in nursing homes and assisted living facilities where residents are often ill and frail and may not have regular visitors. When depression strikes older people, though, its signs are sometimes brushed off as the result of cognitive or age-related changes; grieving, whether normal or complicated, can prompt the same mistake. It's a worrisome fact that suicide risk spikes in older adults, especially among men.

Yet researchers who study grief in older people note certain advantages among people in this age group, too. Tempestuous emotions tend to be damped down, and it's less common for people to respond excitably to worries. Interestingly, research suggests that older adults also have a less intense physiological response to upsetting events. In addition, people often develop better coping strategies as life progresses. One study found that older people were more likely than younger ones to have actively searched for comforting meaning in a death and to have shared this with others.

That said, when a longtime spouse or companion dies, the loss may feel enormous. People who spend many years together develop their own emotional shorthand, language, distinctive roles, and observances. This happens whether or not the relationship is a happy one. When your spouse or partner dies, your identity as half of a couple evaporates, seemingly overnight. You may fit less easily into the lives of friends and be forced to pick up new skills your partner once supplied. Both current and anticipated future loneliness are common. Helplessness, anger, and sometimes even bitterness can arise, as the bereaved person is confronted with new demands and challenges. Friends and family can respond helpfully by listening to, helping, and including the bereaved person,

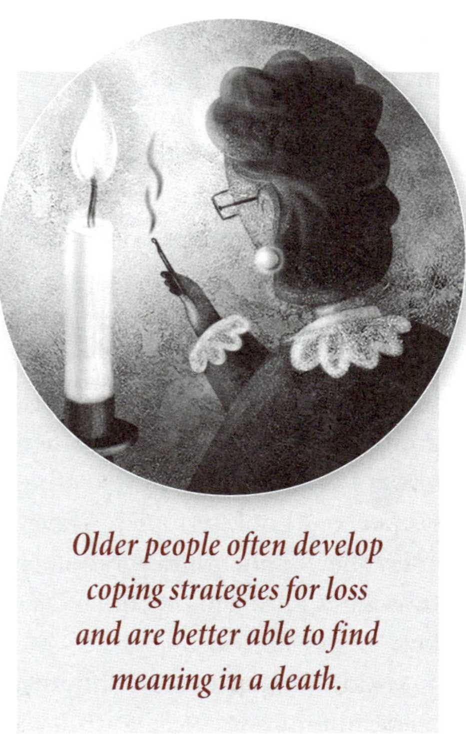

Older people often develop coping strategies for loss and are better able to find meaning in a death.

and by recognizing the existential realities of the bereaved person's situation rather than denying or minimizing it.

It's not only the loss of a spouse that can strike deeply. Almost one in 10 people over 65 has buried a sibling during the previous year. This pain tends to receive little attention, but if you have lost a sibling, you may feel more vulnerable and less resilient. On the other hand, it may also strengthen your ties to your surviving siblings.

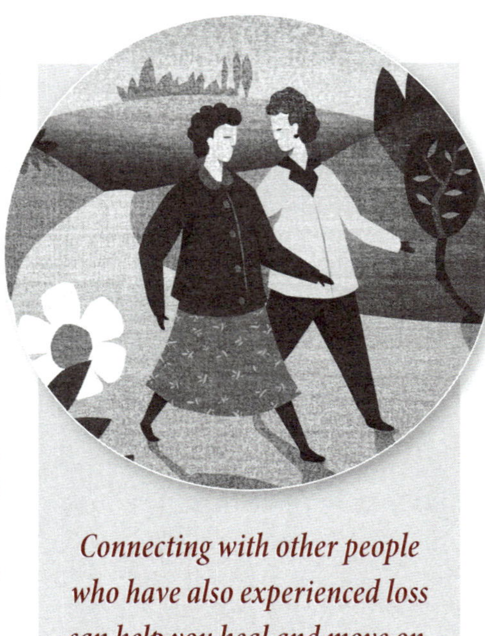

Connecting with other people who have also experienced loss can help you heal and move on.

Reaching out is important

If you're an older adult who is grieving, the strategies suggested in the chapter "Coping with grief and loss" (page 13) can prove helpful. You might also try the following.

Acknowledge your feelings and share them with others. This may help validate your feelings, provide you with emotional support, and alert others to the reality that loss hurts at any age.

Strengthen and broaden your social network. If you have few friends or memberships in community organizations, consider joining a bereavement support group for older people. Many other outlets—ranging from exercise classes and book groups to travel and other opportunities available through a local seniors' organization—can help, too.

Address depression and any suicidal thoughts. Ask your doctor for help, or seek out a mental health professional.

Grief in midlife

The death of a partner requires major adjustments. It's not just the loss of companionship, but a host of other issues as well that come into play.

Whether you're a man or a woman, you're likely to find yourself saddled with a new wave of responsibilities, as you try to fill your partner's roles. Who will provide for the family financially or take care of household chores that your loved one used to handle? How do you fill the emotional void in your children's lives? How do you support the children, when you feel that you are falling apart inside, or worrying about how the family will manage financially? How do you relate as a single person to friends who still are couples?

If you're a parent as well, you face the challenges of simultaneously coping with your own loss and helping the children with theirs, while stabilizing the family, learning new skills, and anticipating a future without the support of a co-parent. Balancing self-care with providing care for the kids is particularly difficult, and you may feel a sense of pressure to be constantly present and constantly vigilant about the children, which can be exhausting and does not leave room for your own healing from grief. Juggling all the responsibilities of midlife—children, jobs, finances, home, other family responsibilities—can be overwhelming.

In other circumstances, if you have been a caregiver for an elderly parent or ailing spouse, a death may offer release from onerous or emotionally painful responsibilities. At the same time, though, it tears the fabric of your daily life and, possibly, severs deep affections and a sense of connection. These conflicting, painful feelings can be hard to wrestle with alone. This is particularly common among women, who are more likely to be caregivers.

But men may suffer their own challenges. Often a grieving widower finds fewer outlets for his grief than a woman in a similar situation. He may feel compelled to hold his emotions inside and reluctant to seek support from friends and from the community. All of these factors can lead to feelings of loneliness and isolation.

Marshalling help

Begin with the strategies in the chapter "Coping with grief and loss" (page 13). In addition, you may find the following suggestions helpful.

Delegate tasks. After a death, many people sincerely offer help but aren't sure what to do. Ask close friends and relatives to step in by helping you plan the funeral or host a gathering afterward. Spell out the tasks that would be most useful—whether handling the phone while you retreat for a while, calling caterers, going along with you to make funeral arrangements, or chauffeuring children or family members. Ask some people if they would be willing to help at a later date; then write down those names and follow up with them. Don't feel guilty. Most people want to help. Capitalize on known strengths—odds are good that you know someone who could help you with financial or legal matters, babysitting, yard work, or jobs around the house.

Set aside time to grieve. Take care of yourself, not just those around you. It is not selfish to need time to grieve or a shoulder to cry on. Often, it helps to hear that others have experienced many of the same feelings—including some emotions we might prefer not to admit to.

Identify people with whom you can safely share your feelings. If no one in your circle fills the bill, consider a bereavement support group or supportive therapist. If you find yourself feeling intensely overwhelmed or depressed, talk with your doctor or a grief counselor or other mental health professional.

Maintain your connections. Men in particular often depend on their spouses for social connection. A new widower may find himself isolated if his spouse took care of maintaining relationships with friends and family. In this situation, finding a therapist or support group and joining some community groups can be helpful. Making a phone list of relatives and friends you can call "to catch up" is also a useful tool. Call one each day.

Get a handle on finances. If finances are a source of anxiety, it's better to address the issue than ignore it. If possible, ask someone to help you. Dig out insurance papers, contact employers, and consider all possible sources of income (see "Gathering essential records," page 11, and "Contacting the appropriate agencies," page 11). With luck, your investigation will reassure you that you needn't immediately take drastic steps, such as selling a house or searching for a new job.

Ask for help. If you find yourself drinking more, using drugs, eating excessively, or engaging in other risky behaviors as you deal with your loss, ask your doctor or a therapist for help. Along with the obvious potential for physical harm, researchers have found that alcohol and drug abuse prolongs distress. Seek help with quitting your use of drugs or alcohol or other self-defeating behaviors through Alcoholics Anonymous or a similar support group.

Grief in children

Children react to loss quite differently from adults. If you could peer inside the minds of children, you would see that their questions, responses, and understanding of death change greatly as they move through different developmental stages. Learning a bit about these changes in development will help you as you guide a child through this difficult time. Take heart: children often are remarkably resilient, and there is much you can do to help them come to terms with their loss and regain joy in life.

Be aware that children normally grieve in fits and spurts. Time out for play or joking may be a much-needed break, rather than a signal that the child has put a loss behind him or her. When a loss is significant—the death of a parent or sibling, especially—a child revisits it repeatedly as he or she grows up. Over time, new layers of its meaning and impact emerge. As a child grows, joyous events, setbacks, and personal triggers for grief sometimes awaken losses presumed to have healed long ago.

Answering kids' top three questions

When someone close is very ill or dies, says the National Cancer Institute, children need a caring answer to three big questions: "Did I cause this death?" "Will it happen to me, too?" "Who is going to care for me?" A child may never ask any of these questions out loud, but you can relieve some pain and fear by bringing up these questions yourself and addressing each one.

What a child age 6 or younger needs

Young children who have lost a loved one are unlikely to fully understand their loss. Providing simple explanations, addressing misconceptions, and offering patient reassurance can help them better understand and cope with their loss.

Offer simple, concrete explanations. What does death mean? Be simple and very concrete. "Uncle Al was so sick that his heart stopped beating and his body stopped working." Or "Death means everything in the body stops—a person doesn't breathe, walk or talk, or feel hungry, sleepy, scared, or sad." Explain that death is permanent, not reversible. Once a person dies, he or she cannot come back to life even though we might wish it.

Try not to use phrasing that could be worrisome or misleading. Saying that "Daddy is sleeping" suggests he'll wake up, and it equates a normal, everyday activity with death. Stating that "We lost Aunt Emily" implies she can be found or that the child, too, could be lost. "God took Jimmy early because he was so good" might raise many concerns, rather than soothe a sore heart.

Reassure your child. If Daddy died young, will Mommy die, too? This was a question Sheryl Sandberg faced after her husband's sudden death, leaving her with two young children. "[A social worker] advised me not to make a false promise to them that I would live forever," she writes in *Option B*, "but rather explain to them that it was very unusual for someone to die so young. Mostly she told me to say over and over that I loved them and we would get through this together."

Address magical thinking. Children this age often engage in magical thinking. They may worry that they provoked the death with an angry thought or outburst ("I hate you! I wish you'd die!"). Or they may believe there was something they could have done to prevent the death. Reassure your child that nothing he or she did or didn't do caused the death. You might say, "Some children believe something they did made a death happen. You may worry that something you said or did caused Mommy to die. It's not true. Mommy died because she was very, very sick. Nothing you did, said, or thought made her sick."

Be patient with repetition. Children may ask the same questions over and over as they try to form a concept of death. Patiently answering questions—even those that seem upsetting or repetitious—helps them to do so.

What a child age 7 to 12 needs

Slightly older children who have lost a parent need to know that, despite the loss, life will continue in a safe and normal pattern—that they will be cared for. They may need reassurance that they are not to blame, as well as comfort and support. Older children also need a fuller explanation of the death.

Offer more information. A child this age may want to know more details: "What was wrong with Dad's heart? How did the doctors try to fix it? Where is his body now?" She or he can grasp the concept that death is permanent and may have many questions. Be guided by these questions in choosing what information to offer.

Provide reassurance. Just as younger children need to hear that they didn't cause the death, so, too, do children this age. Remind them of all the things that will not change—their friends at school, their classes, their sports, their house, the rest of the family. Don't be afraid to continue activities that you all did together as a family.

Be a good listener. Children may have many more questions than they openly ask, especially if they're worried about upsetting you. Tell them it's okay to ask about anything, even questions that seem silly or dumb. You might ask other caring adults to do the same.

What a teenager needs

Teens often turn to their friends for solace, but they will still need reassurance, answers to questions, and comfort from family.

Let them ask questions and share feelings. Teens are not yet adults, although some try to act very mature. Listen closely. Offer hugs. While remembering that teens are still young, be willing to share information when they ask questions, and involve them with decisions about services and funerals.

Reassure them. Teens also need reminders that nothing they did—or didn't do—caused the death. Adolescence is a time to separate from parents, but this normal need for independence can complicate grieving. The desire for independence may have prompted conflicts. Once again, reassure a teen that any harsh words spoken ("I wish you'd die!") didn't cause the death, and that their loved one understood that the teen loved him or her. A parent's death can be especially hard at this time, because the teen may feel guilty for having pushed away emotionally from the parent and have strong conflicting feelings.

Talk about the future. Teens may have financial fears or worries about future plans. Gently expressing and exploring these issues may be worthwhile.

Give them a chance to be with their tribe. Often, teens want to talk to and spend time with friends. Grieving together can be an enormous solace.

Expect conflict. Teenagers, especially older teenagers, are struggling to separate and define themselves as independent of their parents. When a parent dies, they are thrust back into a more vulnerable position, or may feel needed at home in a new way. It is not uncommon for a teenager to feel conflict about being with family and being with friends, and this can sometimes play out as anger or avoidance of the family.

For all children

At every age, children need hugs and affection. You can also do the following to help children grieve.

Allow children to safely express emotions. Sadness, tears, laughter, hurt, anger, relief—try to let your child share her or his feelings with you.

Consider what lies beneath. Bravado, obnoxious jokes or behavior, aggressiveness, clinginess, irritability, or apparent indifference can all be expressions of a child's grief. Some children try to comfort others by setting aside their own needs or acting perfect or like little adults. Others would rather make you angry than see you sad.

Offer reassurance. In the wake of any tragedy, children worry about what will happen to them. Tell children that they are loved and will be cared for.

Try to limit secondary losses. Moving, experiencing the fallout of financial setbacks, and not having someone cheering in the bleachers or attending school events are all examples of secondary losses. Whenever possible, try to preserve a child's routine and recognize feelings that arise as a result of unavoidable changes.

Play together and openly encourage joy. If you're grieving, this advice may seem impossible. But remember, a child needs to know it's acceptable to take a break from grief, to have fun again, and to spend loving time in your presence. Let the child be a kid.

Don't be afraid to talk about the departed. Even if your loved one is gone, he or she is still an important person in your child's life story. Let the child know about all the things that made your loved one unique. In addition to the major accomplishments, be sure to include the quirky details—how he or she traveled thousands of miles one year to see a solar eclipse, or restored vintage cars, or was transformed by becoming a parent—and just how proud he or she was of that child. Continue to do things that you all enjoyed doing together as a family. You are still a family, though a smaller one, and it's important to honor that.

Bereavement programs for families help many children whose mothers or fathers die. It's not yet clear which children and adolescents are likely to benefit most or which programs are best. One study suggested those who were at higher risk—for example, because of a suicide of a loved one or because they exhibited greater distress—benefited from intervention.

Preparing children for a funeral

When it comes to involvement in a funeral or memorial service, be guided by the child. Some people feel it helps to involve the child in planning for services. Understand, though, that funerals and other rituals can be frightening to a child.

No child should go to a funeral without being prepared for what will happen. Before the service, describe the rituals and sights that a child will see there. Share what the room will look like, who will be there, how they might feel and act, and what the child will see. If the casket will be open, explain how the deceased will look. Also, ask the child how he or she might like to say goodbye. Encourage children to commemorate the person who died in a way that feels meaningful to them. Writing a poem or song, drawing, or doing something the deceased enjoyed can be satisfying to a child.

If a child doesn't want to attend a funeral or service, ask what's worrying him or her and what would help. Try to soothe fears while still answering honestly. Most experts believe that it's best not to force a reluctant child to participate. When children do wish to participate, it helps to assign an adult to act as a buddy at the service. That way, if a child becomes overwhelmed or wants to leave, someone is available to help take him or her outside or to a quiet place. Ideally, this shouldn't be a loved one who wishes to stay at the service.

Losing a child

Surviving a child's death has been described by many people as the worst pain of all. Grieving is often intense and prolonged, whether the child died young or much later in life.

It's easy to intuit what makes this loss so difficult and different from others. A child represents his or her parents, the future, the hopes and dreams and fulfillment of deeply held needs and longings; a young child's vulnerability and dependency may contribute to a feeling of failure for parents. The strong attachment to the child, so necessary for the child's healthy growth, may also intensify the grieving process. The death of a child violates a natural order of life—that older people die before younger ones. The loss of a child represents the loss of part of the self, and profoundly disrupts a family. It destroys future possibilities, and the continuity conferred as one generation passes its values, experiences, and genes to the next is lost. It severs deeply wired biological and emotional ties. It can irrevocably shake religious beliefs and assumptions about how the world works.

The age of a child may make a difference in the twists grief takes. While many parents fulfill the role of nurturer all of their lives, the defining tasks and routines are strongest while children are young. Virtually every aspect of life is steeped in moment-to-moment reminders of the loss of a young child. When an adult child dies, a parent's daily routine may be less affected, but other unsettling realities may appear. Previously hidden aspects of the child's life that come to light may be distressing. Ties with grandchildren may be weakened as the surviving spouse moves on with life or remarries. Parents may feel abandoned, and lose the security of knowing they have a child to care for them in the future.

The grief for the loss of a child never completely goes away, and the grieving process immediately after the death is often more intense and prolonged than after the death of a partner or spouse. Parents may feel especially isolated from those whose children are healthy and alive, and social networks may be constricted. Young parents, especially, may lack the mature coping mechanisms and communities that help people through the grieving process. A central part of grieving is making meaning of the death, and parents may struggle to find any sense of meaning in such a cruel loss; others may construct meaning in a religious framework, and still others will find ways of creating meaning through renewed or enhanced focus on other children or other activities.

While most parents, over time, are able to cope with the death of a child, the parents of young children who die are at elevated risk for complicated grief, depression, suicide, and medical problems. Mothers, in particular, are at high risk, as are parents whose children died suddenly or unexpectedly, those who lose an only child, and those who perceive their child to have had a difficult end-of-life care experience.

Although there are often two parents grieving the death of a child, people grieve this terrible loss differently. In some circumstances, these different approaches to grieving may strengthen the parental unit; in others, these differences may prevent parents from comforting each other, and may even cause strife and distance. One parent may feel angry with the other because of a lack of support or the perception that the other doesn't care enough or seems out of control. If one of the parents was in some way responsible for the child's death, the anger and isolation can be even deeper. The death can be so overwhelming that it's sometimes impossible to lean upon each other.

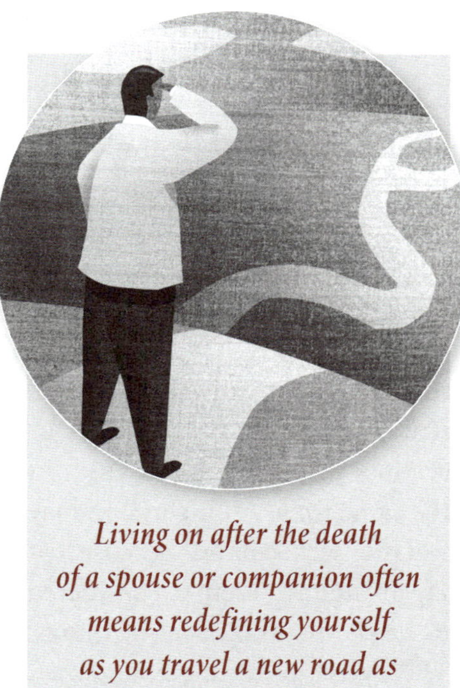

Living on after the death of a spouse or companion often means redefining yourself as you travel a new road as a single person.

If a married adult child dies, a parent may find it painful to realize that he or she is not next of kin and has less control over decisions that follow in the wake of the death. And the loss of support to aged parents that an adult child can supply will also be missed.

Advice for grieving parents

Nothing can bring a child back, of course, and the pain is never entirely erased. However, the suggestions below, as well as some of the strategies from "Coping with grief and loss" (page 13) may offer some solace.

Create a meaningful memorial. Planting a tree, making donations to children's hospitals and medical research, or committing to a cause such as preventing drunk driving (see "A good cause," page 20) are a few examples. You might even establish a scholarship fund or charitable foundation in your child's name.

Seek support. Research shows that support from others, self-help groups, and counseling or psychotherapy can help parents come to terms with their loss. Family bereavement counseling can be especially important when other children are affected by the death or when spouses deal with their grief very differently. If stress and grief have frayed your connection to your partner, couples therapy may be helpful to you as you try to rebuild those bonds.

Mourn every loss. Stillbirths, miscarriages, and infertility are examples of losses that often are not mourned publicly. Even close friends and family may not understand the impact of the loss unless it's explained to them. Acknowledge and mourn the loss.

Allow yourself to continue your relationship with your child. Although nothing can bring back a child who has died, parents who allow themselves to forge a sense of continued connection with their child may fare better during bereavement. Give yourself permission to remember, to imagine what your child would be like at different ages and stages, to recognize and acknowledge what would be meaningful moments in the life of the child you lost.

Losing a parent

The death of a parent is another profound loss at any age. When it occurs during childhood, its echoes reverberate throughout the rest of your life. According to many experts, children whose parents die revisit their loss and grieve anew as developmental stages unfold. Likewise, the absence of a parent at important moments—whether it's a ball game or spelling bee, college graduation, marriage, or a baby's birth—continually underscores the loss.

Children who have reached adulthood may be more mature, but they face their own challenges in coping with the death of a parent. The death of a parent thrusts adult children into new roles. It forces them to consider an identity separate from being a son or a daughter and challenges them to examine their own lives. It may also cause them to reflect on the nature of their relationships with their parents, their siblings, and other family members. Young adult children face the challenges of parenting, juggling work and home responsibilities, and achieving independence and creating a life for themselves, without the guidance, support, and security that a parent can provide.

Later in life, the death of a parent can have still other meanings. It raises uncomfortable questions of mortality and responsibility. Ready or not, the survivor may now be the family matriarch or patriarch. It reconfigures relationships among survivors, particularly if a parent was the emotional glue that held the family together. It severs ties to the past and crushes the illusion, if not reality, of a warm sanctuary in a sometimes cold world. At the same time, adult children may feel they lack support, because losing an elderly parent is considered to be the natural order of things. The sense of being abandoned and adrift without support can be powerful.

Not every parent-child relationship is a warm one, of course. And often, when a parent had a lingering illness or Alzheimer's disease, caregivers may feel released to go on with their own lives. But such difficulties or outright conflicts between parent and child don't necessarily make grieving easier.

Advice if you've lost a parent

If you have lost a parent, some of the strategies suggested below may prove comforting.

Acknowledge submerged feelings. Sometimes, family members resurrect old hurts and patterns after a death. Planning a funeral and distributing belongings can be flash points (see "Understand that personal items may hold special meaning for others," page 17). Try your best to communicate and avoid misunderstandings.

Pass the baton. Ask the youngest family member at holiday gatherings to say a blessing once given by your parent, or ask everyone to join in.

Plan for difficult days. Mother's Day, Father's Day, birthdays, and other family holidays can be especially painful. Plan an outing your loved one would have enjoyed or a commemorative activity.

Find other parental figures. Although a parent who has died cannot be replaced, other relationships with people like your parent, in age, interests, or personality, can help re-establish a connection with some of the qualities of the person who died. Such relationships can be a source of ongoing support and nurturance after a parent is gone.

Losing a spouse or life partner

Living on after a spouse or companion dies is a tough trek. In a single stroke, you may find that dreams of the future and the repository of your shared past have been swept away. Responsibilities easily juggled by two can overwhelm one, especially with grief and the needs of any children piled on top. A plummeting income or the need to search for work can add further stress.

In general, the intensity of grief fades over time. As noted earlier, grief is not a linear process; there is no right way or correct timeline for grieving. Some people assume that by a few weeks after a loss, the bereaved spouse should be "ready to move on." By contrast, in some cultures, ongoing grief and the external expressions of bereavement ("widow's weeds") are expected forever.

In this culture, by six months after the loss of a partner, most people are beginning to heal. However, the processes of grieving, re-creating a life of one's own, and finding a personal identity apart from the person who has died usually take considerably longer. While many bereaved people are adjusting well by several months after the death of a partner, there is tremendous variation. In particular, highly dependent relationships create challenges in the grieving process, as the person left behind needs to find new sources of support, as well as new practical coping mechanisms.

There are other potential complications. Any ambivalence or conflict that existed in the relationship can force the bereaved person to hold big contradictions in mind as he or she processes the loss. Many of the particulars lost—the sexual intimacy, the small private rituals and stories that many couples create, the presence of a daily partner to share meals and experiences—can be difficult to explain to others, adding to a sense of isolation. Developing new networks, activities, and patterns often takes months or years. However, people metabolize grief differently, and some people move through grief as they return to work or develop new relationships.

A study in the *Journal of Personality and Social Psychology* looked at a national sampling of more than 750 men and women after the death of a spouse. The researchers found that even decades after the death, partners still talked, thought, and felt emotion about the deceased. Generally, upsetting thoughts declined over time, while thoughts prompting happier feelings did not. Anniversary reactions—that is, painful thoughts about the loss or distress at reminders—tended to occur at least sometimes and feel somewhat intense for seven to eight years after the loss. Less frequently, these reactions still cropped up decades later. The researchers noted perceptions of personal growth and greater self-confidence, too.

Figure 1: Widows and widowers

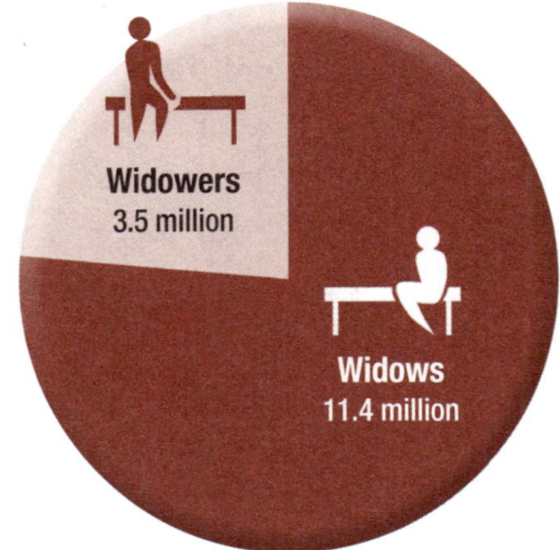

There are nearly 15 million widows and widowers in the United States. Women are more likely than men to suffer the loss of a spouse; in fact, there are more than three times as many widows (11.4 million) as there are widowers (3.5 million) in this country.

Source: U.S. Census Bureau, 2016.

Starting to rebuild your life

The strategies described earlier may help. In addition, try these.

Find appropriate support. Your age, sexual identity, and life experiences may shape your needs. Find a support group that is geared for you; there are groups for young widows, widowed parents, older spouses, and gays or lesbians. If appropriate, find solace with others who have had someone they love die through violent trauma or after lengthy illness. If necessary, do not be ashamed to seek counseling.

Try not to blame yourself. There are always things you could have done differently. No one has perfect foresight as to how events will unfold. You did your best with the imperfect knowledge you had at the time. Also, if you were not there when your loved one died, realize that most people aren't.

Build your skills. Long-term relationships encourage division of tasks, such as cooking, driving, home repair, child care, and managing family finances. The lack of certain skills can feed your anxiety and feelings of helplessness. Once you've identified the gaps, however, you'll probably find that you are capable of learning these skills—and that sense of accomplishment, in turn, can help build your confidence in other areas of your life.

When a loved one has a life-threatening illness

Most people who pick up this report are looking for solace following a devastating loss. However, some readers are anticipating a loss. They, too, are grieving, though the quality of that grief is different. If you are caring for someone you love at the end of his or her life, we hope that this chapter will help you ease the burden.

Time seems to freeze when you learn that someone you love has a life-threatening illness. Maybe you instinctively push the news away. Or perhaps you cry, or swing into action. No matter what happens that day or over the ensuing months or years, time and life go on after the diagnosis is made, regardless of whether you feel ready to cope. Inevitably, you start confronting the possibility of loss before it actually happens.

The course of life-threatening illnesses can vary, of course. You and your loved one may pursue promising treatments and perhaps enjoy a respite from encroaching mortality. Some people with life-threatening illnesses are cured. But in other cases, the illness progresses or re-emerges, and your loved one's health keeps declining. Even as treatments are still ongoing, there is a great deal you can do to make this a meaningful time for both of you.

Some of the support you need is emotional, and the fears and feelings that surface now are better aired than ignored. You may also need help with practical details, including help arranging to make medical decisions when your loved one is unable to do so. This chapter can guide you through some of these steps and suggest additional resources for you to draw on. It can also help you assist your loved one who is facing a life-threatening illness.

As the illness unfolds: Worry, sadness, and grief

Living with a life-threatening illness means living with loss, for both you and your loved one. Blows to independence and security, impaired abilities, and truncated visions of the future are just a few examples of the losses that arise in this setting. Compounding all of these is the uncertainty of what lies ahead. But remember that living, even in the shadow of death, is still living, and there are opportunities for growth, connection, and emotional healing. Following are some strategies for making the most of this time.

Focus on your most important goals and priorities. Whether days, weeks, months, or years remain, it's important for both of you to think about your goals during this period. Focusing on personal goals can be a way of warding off despair and hopelessness. Moreover, if energy is limited, it is essential to use it for what really matters.

For most people, spending time with family and friends is even more important than it has been; sometimes, trade-offs need to be made to allow for that time. This might entail reducing commitments to work, or deciding not to spend time with people with whom you are less connected. If medical treatments are crowding out all other activities, see if you can reorganize appointments and treatments in a way that minimizes their interference with your loved one's goals. You can ask the doctor about a "vacation" from treatments, if you wish. These shifts in priorities can help you and your loved one make the most of your remaining time together.

Focus on what's possible. Maybe certain goals are no longer attainable. Try adjusting the goals rather than abandoning them. Say your daughter is expecting a baby six months from now, and from the doctor's prognosis, you know it's unlikely your loved one will be alive to see your new grandchild. Maybe the two of you can help prepare the nursery or have an early baby shower. In this way, it's still possible for your loved one to share in the joy of the upcoming birth.

Do it now. If there's something that's important to both of you, do it now rather than putting it off, even if you have to downsize your goals. For example, if you've always dreamed of taking a trip to Iceland together, take it if you can. But if failing health makes that impossible, plan a special activity that's closer to home.

Live in the moment. If you take that trip, try to savor every minute. Create good memories for yourself that will help see you through rough times ahead. Even when your loved one is confined to a hospital bed, you may find that there are moments to cherish—for example, if you hold meaningful conversations, reminisce about good times, and express love and appreciation, as well as forgiveness for any past hurts (see "Sharing love and letting go," page 42).

Let your loved one teach you. A person with a serious illness frequently feels helpless. Being able to impart useful information helps counter the sense of diminishment that comes with an illness, and can be therapeutic for the person who is sick. Ask him or her about practical things—where the key to the safe deposit box is kept, for example, or how to make a favorite family recipe. Encourage your loved one to share important values and beliefs about how to live a good life. Letting the person teach you gives your loved one a sense of continued purpose, and can also give *you* useful information and a sense of being loved and cared for.

Acknowledge the uncertainty. Most family members continue to hope for a good outcome, and those hopes and wishes may make it hard to see what truly lies ahead. But at some point, you need to prepare for the possibility that things won't turn out the way you hope. Talking about and making plans for the eventuality that your loved one may not survive does not mean that hope is gone or that you are giving up. Rather, it will help you support your loved one in case things go poorly, and help you be prepared for what comes. You may have worries about how to cope when you're alone, or feelings of being abandoned. These are normal.

Discuss important questions. Your loved one needs to tell you what type of care he or she wants as the illness continues to unfold. Here are some of the questions that should be addressed:

- If time is short, how do you want to spend your remaining days, weeks, or months?
- What are you willing to go through for the chance of having more time?
- What is so essential to your well-being that you wouldn't want to be without it?
- If you get sicker, where do you want to be? Home? Hospital?
- What are your fears and worries about what is ahead?
- How will you talk with your kids about your illness?
- How do you make sure your family's needs are honored?
- How much suffering do you expect?
- How much pain is too much pain?
- Do you want treatment aimed at keeping you alive as long as possible, regardless of the side effects? Or do you want to focus on comfort in your last days?

While your loved one may have already addressed some of these issues in an advance directive (see "Advance care directives," page 36), such questions will need to be revisited over time. That's because the answers may change as your loved one gets sicker.

Talking about the future, including death

No matter what role you play in your loved one's care, talking with him or her about the future, including death, is important, albeit difficult. Possibly you worry that you'll undercut your loved one's will to continue or that you'll increase his or her fears. Simply raising the possibility that the illness may get worse may seem like a form of abandonment because it suggests you've given up on the lingering promise of a cure. Your own anxiety, sadness, and discomfort may make the words choke in your throat.

Yet most people who are confronting a challenging situation find comfort in sharing concerns, having an opportunity to prepare, and thinking through tough decisions that they might face in the future. These early conversations, difficult as they are, will help you both to face harder times, when they come.

Raising these issues can help in multiple ways. It is often easier to address the topics than it is to keep up a good front and carry on conversations that strike false notes. For most people, "unspeakable" issues are the most frightening, and opening the door to talking about them makes them less scary. Airing your concerns can also relieve loneliness, making you and your loved one feel closer, and can allow you to share your strength and courage.

You may also find that your loved one has been stifling numerous fears—such as the fear of leaving friends and family, losing control, becoming a burden, and leaving tasks and plans unfinished. Many people dread a painful death. Sharing such fears and expressing beliefs about death can help people feel less overwhelmed. Talking can help reduce some of the sadness and anxiety that people with serious illnesses inevitably experience. It can also diminish physical pain, which is aggravated by fear.

Preparing for this difficult conversation

Clearly, not everyone who is seriously ill is ready to talk about death. So how will you know when to talk and what to say? Below are some ideas that may help you. Your task in this difficult time is merely to open the door to this conversation and promise to stay for it, if the person you care for wishes to talk.

Look for openings. A sermon or song you heard, a book you read, or the way someone else's illness and death unfolded can be an opportunity for remarks that open the door. By commenting, you signal that you're ready to talk and needn't be protected.

Broach the topic gently. Elisabeth Kübler-Ross, psychiatrist and author of the book *On Death and Dying*, describes conversations with dying people that start with the simplest question: "How sick are you?" Other questions you can ask are "What do you worry about?" "How can I help?" "Is there anything you want to talk about?" Try not to rebuff tentatively expressed fears with hearty assurances, such as "That's a long way off" or "Of course you're not a burden." It might help instead to ask more specifically, "What are you thinking about?" If your loved one is receptive to talking about these issues, you may wish to open the door to questions like "How you would like to be cared for as you get sicker?" and "How much do you find yourself thinking about death?" Sharing your own thoughts may help.

Let it go. Kübler-Ross notes that people slip into and out of denial during the course of illness and even during a single conversation. Denial is a normal and healthy way of dealing with a serious illness. Sometimes it's too hard to think or talk about death. Let your loved one end conversations that feel too difficult. Allow him or her to hold on to comforting thoughts and fantasies, as long as they are not getting in the way of getting good health care, taking care of necessary tasks, and being close to others.

Planning for a funeral or memorial service

Funerals and memorial services may seem like bleak or sorrowful subjects. Yet discussing these matters with a person who has a serious illness may help relieve concerns. Such conversations can also offer comforting guidance for the survivors. Of course, not everyone has the opportunity or the desire to discuss these issues. It is important to remember that funerals and memorial services are for the people who remain behind, and that, in most situations, your loved one would want you to do what feels right to you.

Some people feel comforted by talking about funeral and memorial plans while they're alive. Squaring away details—what it will cost, how to pay, what shape a service or memorial should take, what sort of casket to buy, what music might be played, and who should speak—may alleviate worries. It can also be a chance for you and your loved one to express your feelings about each other and the time you shared. Consider gently raising the topic with a person who is seriously ill: "I want to do whatever would feel right for you after you are gone. Would you like to talk about planning for a funeral or memorial service?"

Advance care directives

Ideally, your loved one will be able to make all the decisions about his or her medical care right up until the end, retaining control over that care. Advance care directives are designed for the situation in which the person can no longer communicate. An advance care directive helps ensure that your loved one's health care wishes and end-of-life concerns are known and respected. These documents address how aggressively doctors should pursue life-sustaining measures and how to balance quality of life and comfort in making treatment choices. The ideal time to do this is before these issues become pressing.

Health care power of attorney

Your loved one should have a durable power of attorney for health care naming a person to serve as health care proxy and should communicate to the designated proxy his or her personal values about care. These are the types of questions you should ask your loved one to answer:

- If you had severe brain damage, would you want to be kept alive by machines, such as a mechanical ventilator, and to receive artificial hydration and nutrition (tube feeding)? (For definitions of these terms, see "Life support measures," at right.)
- If you were unable to breathe on your own, would you want to be kept alive by a mechanical ventilator for a trial period if your doctor thought it might help you regain consciousness? Would you want it stopped if it failed to help?
- If medical care appears unlikely to extend meaningful life, would you want other treatments to be stopped and comfort care begun in order to relieve pain, labored breathing, nausea, anxiety, confusion, and other distressing symptoms?
- Do you have any religious or spiritual beliefs that should guide doctors and others responsible for making decisions about your care?
- Would you like to be an organ and tissue donor (see "Organ and tissue donation," page 38)?

Talking with your loved one about his or her wishes for end-of-life care is one of the most important steps you can take to ensure that you are doing the right thing, should your loved one be unable to make these decisions at the end. This is good not only for your loved one, but also for you, as it relieves you of the burden of making tough decisions without adequate information. And knowing your loved one's wishes can help alleviate your guilt and regret about those decisions, if you should ultimately have to make the very difficult decision to withdraw life support.

State laws vary, so it is important to make sure any advance directive complies with local regulations. A local hospital, hospice, or seniors' organization may have staff members who can help prepare an advance directive. Or discuss this with a lawyer qualified in elder law. (It's wise for everyone to have advance directives, so you and other adult family members should consider preparing them as well.)

Advance directives have some major flaws, including the impossibility of knowing the exact circumstances under which they will be invoked, what medical options will be available, and how the person's feelings might have changed in the interim. Nonetheless, thinking about and talking about care wishes for various circumstances can help everyone sort out values and feelings about medical measures often taken at the end of life. Moreover, the closer you are to the decisions that are likely to arise because of known health problems, the more specific you can be in the instructions. A frank talk with a doctor about possible medical scenarios can provide guidance. Your loved one's wishes should be communicated fully with everyone involved, and conversations about treatment should be revisited whenever medical circumstances change.

If your loved one has a life-threatening illness, it's important to take the following steps:

Life support measures

It is difficult to predict these things in advance, but it's worth considering whether you will or won't want the following life support options (once again, bear in mind that your spoken wishes override any written ones):

Mechanical ventilation: A machine called a ventilator or respirator forces air into the lungs for people who are unable to breathe under their own power.

Intravenous hydration: A tube inserted into a vein supplies a solution of water, sugar, and minerals for people who are unable to swallow.

Artificial nutrition (tube feeding): A tube inserted into the stomach through the nose (short-term) or abdomen (longer-term) supplies nutrients and fluids for people who are unable to swallow.

Hemodialysis: Blood is circulated through a machine to maintain the balance of fluids and essential minerals and clear waste from the bloodstream for people whose kidneys are unable to perform this function.

- Make sure that anyone named as proxy in a durable power of attorney for health care has a copy of the advance directive and knows your loved one's goals for medical care. The proxy, a family member, and a lawyer, if any, should know where additional copies of the form are kept.
- Talk with your loved one's doctors to be sure the wishes are understood and can be followed. Ask the staff to place a copy of the advance directive in your loved one's permanent medical record.
- Discuss wishes for end-of-life medical care with family members, so that everyone is on the same page if decisions need to be made later. Acknowledge that this is a difficult topic. It may help to begin by talking about the end-of-life treatment of another close relative or friend.
- Have discussions with family and medical staff more than once to be sure wishes are understood. Try to do this as circumstances change.

Organ and tissue donation

Depending on your loved one's cause of death, organ and tissue donation may be possible. Sometimes the knowledge that one's organs can bring life or health to someone else later is quite meaningful to the person who is dying as well as to family members.

Next of kin must consent to organ donation after a death, so be sure that the person explains his or her wishes to family members and doctors. In some cases, a home death would make organ and tissue donation impossible.

For more information, check with the United Network for Organ Sharing at www.unos.org or 888-894-6361 (toll-free).

Orders for life-sustaining treatment (POLST, MOLST, POST, or MOST)

Physician orders for life-sustaining treatment (POLST)—also known in different states as medical orders for life-sustaining treatment (MOLST), physician orders for scope of treatment (POST), or medical orders for scope of treatment (MOST)—are increasingly being used to guide care for those with advanced illness in the event that they are unable to speak for themselves. These forms give your loved one's wishes the authority of a physician-written medical order that is portable and effective across care settings. Thus, his or her wishes can guide treatment in an emergency—in the hospital, at a nursing facility, or at home. That's not the case with standard advance directives, which typically are not binding in emergency situations where a doctor's orders are essential.

According the National POLST Paradigm Task Force, these medical orders are most appropriate for people who have serious, life-limiting illnesses, or who are significantly weakened and experience extreme difficulty with daily tasks because of advanced frailty. POLST and similar forms spell out goals for care and level of treatment desired, and they do this using concrete orders that enable emergency personnel and physicians to take action. The questions they cover are similar to those for the health care power of attorney. For example, do you want comfort care measures only (such as pain relief, wound care, and oxygen if needed for comfort)? Do you want full medical treatment (for example, mechanical ventilation and a variety of medications)? Would you want short-term or long-term artificial nutrition or no artificial nutrition at all? Would you want CPR to be attempted if your heart stops beating?

POLST/MOLST forms

- are written by a doctor or health care provider after consulting with the person (or, possibly, with family members or a chosen surrogate if the person is incapacitated)
- reflect your loved one's preferences for current and future care, unless he or she changes or voids the POLST/MOLST form
- complement but do not replace any additional instructions offered by a health care proxy
- can be shared through electronic medical records
- can be posted at home for emergency medical personnel (usually on the refrigerator) or carried with your loved one
- can always be revised if circumstances or wishes change.

At this writing, all states except South Dakota, Michigan, and Arkansas have a POLST, MOLST, POST, or MOST program or are developing one.

Do-not-resuscitate orders

A do-not-resuscitate order (DNR) tells health care professionals not to attempt cardiopulmonary resuscitation (CPR) or defibrillation if the person's heart stops beating. It is also referred to as a "no code," a do-not-attempt-resuscitation order (DNAR), or an allow-natural-death order (AND). This document is written to cover circumstances in which such measures are unlikely to revive the person or prolong meaningful life. It's worth noting that health care and emergency personnel will presume your loved one wants CPR if there is no DNR or POLST form, even if he or she has asked family members to forgo this measure. Even with a DNR, it will not hold in the home, unless you have a "non-hospital DNR" or "out-of-hospital DNR," which may be represented by a DNR bracelet that EMS personnel will recognize and honor.

Why would anyone want a DNR? If a person has a terminal illness or little hope of improving enough to continue a life that's meaningful, he or she may wish to let nature take its course rather than having CPR. CPR is very often not successful and is physically traumatic—for example, ribs may be broken, and intubation to provide mechanical breathing is common.

Discuss the need for a DNR with your family and doctors. It may be reassuring to know that even with a DNR, your loved one will continue to receive appropriate medical care to treat short-term illnesses or injuries and relieve pain or other troubling symptoms. Emergency service personnel called to your home can still give oxygen, medications, and fluids and transport the person to a hospital, if necessary.

There are different types of DNR orders, and forms and laws vary from state to state, so it's important to discuss this with your loved one's physician. Generally, only original documents are valid, so it's wise to have several original copies of a DNR form. Always keep one handy in your loved one's home; you or a caregiver should carry the other at all times. In hospitals and nursing homes, the DNR is kept on file and noted in your loved one's chart. Mistakes do occur, so ask if this has been done.

Most states are now replacing DNRs with POLST (MOLST, POST, or MOST), which include CPR as one option that can be accepted or rejected.

Caregiver stress

Anticipation of the end can be especially intense for those who are full-time caregivers. The Family Caregiver Alliance estimates that upward of 20% of family caregivers suffer from depression, twice the rate of the general population. And former caregivers may continue to experience distress even after caregiving ends. One study found that 41% of former caregivers of a spouse with Alzheimer's disease or another form of dementia experienced mild to severe depression up to three years after their spouse had died.

Researchers have linked caregiving to a greater risk of high blood pressure, sluggish wound healing, and other signs of a distressed immune system, as well as self-reports of poor health. Certainly, when caregivers are exhausted, stressed, and isolated, their health suffers. But the culprit isn't merely caregiving, which can forge a loving, healthy connection. It's the difficulty of finding the time to eat well, exercise, enjoy life, release stress, and get the rest and support you need when you're caring for someone around the clock or combining care with an already full plate.

It is also important to acknowledge that some caregiving experiences are extremely challenging, because of strain, abuse, or hurts in the past relationship, anger and recrimination from the person who is ill, and the sheer difficulties of providing care. Finding a support system is particularly important under these circumstances.

Steps for easing caregiver stress

To provide the best care you can for your loved one at this difficult time, start with yourself. In addition to eating well and exercising most days, try to do some of the following:

Tackle stress head-on. When stress has no outlet, it compounds quickly. Has your confused father asked why he can't go back home for the 10th time in as many minutes? Have medical appointments compelled you to miss work again? Are you worried about paying soaring prescription drug bills? Clearly, you cannot completely erase sources of stress in your life. But you can relieve some stress and work on solutions to problems that are filling your days with stress. Take a time-out: listen to music you like, enjoy a luxurious bath, take a yoga class, dabble in art or creative pastimes, go out to dinner, or splurge on a massage. Regular time off helps make the point that you're neither invincible nor completely irreplaceable.

Retrench. Reassess needs and brainstorm solutions. Would adult day services help once or twice a week? Would grocery shopping online give you a little more time for yourself? Can other family members step up to the plate or pitch in financially?

Release feelings. Sometimes stress stems from feelings you wish you didn't have, such as anger, frustration, or dislike. Find ways to release these feelings without hurting yourself or others. Talk with understanding friends, or consider therapy. Yell in the car with the windows rolled up. Sprint up and down the stairs to burn energy.

Relax. Learn meditation and other relaxation techniques through a class, CD, DVD, or book. The time and money invested pay dividends in improved health and well-being.

Talk with a mental health clinician (social worker, psychologist, or psychiatrist). Dealing with a loved one's illness is stressful and can trigger feelings of anxiety, depression, loneliness, guilt, and sorrow. It can help to have a place to share these feelings, gain perspective, learn skills for coping with stress and grief, and mobilize your inner resources to take care of yourself and your loved one. When you are in the midst of caregiving, it is easy to lose perspective; a counselor can provide support, another viewpoint, and expertise in helping you cope with the challenges of caregiving and anticipated loss.

Talk with your religious leader, or a hospice or hospital chaplain. Priests, rabbis, and other religious leaders can offer real comfort to believers. Even people who do not regularly attend religious services may turn toward their faith as an illness progresses.

Talk to someone who's been there. Seek out sympathetic friends or family who have weathered similar situations.

Talking with the treatment team

It's important during this time to keep channels of communication open with your loved one's doctors. A physician's knowledge about how the illness might progress and how pain will be handled can be invaluable. A study in *Archives of Internal Medicine* by doctors at Harvard Medical School and the Dana-Farber Cancer Institute found that relationships with doctors can play a significant role in how people who are seriously ill view their quality of life—even when recovery is not possible. "When medicine is no longer able to cure, physicians may still positively and significantly influence the lives of their patients," wrote Holly Prigerson, lead author of the study and an expert on bereavement and end-of-life care. "By reducing patient worry, encouraging contemplation, integrating pastoral care within medical care, fostering a therapeutic alliance between patient and physician that enables patients to feel dignified, and preventing unnecessary hospitalizations and receipt of life-prolonging care, clinicians can enable their patients to live their last days with the highest possible level of comfort and care."

Realize, though, that it's not unusual for doctors (and nurses) to shy away from talking about death. Some view death as a failure and feel determined to try everything to prevent it. Being human, they have their own fears and discomfort to deal with, too.

Sometimes, when the doctor is reluctant, it is necessary for you to initiate the conversation. It is entirely appropriate for you to bring up your questions with the doctors. Your loved one may not be able to speak for him or herself, and you need to be your loved one's voice. Rather than feeling abandoned, most patients with serious illnesses find it helpful to have information about what is likely to happen. Most people want to know about time, so that they can make decisions and prioritize important personal goals.

Physicians often wait until you give a clue that you are ready to discuss end-of-life issues before broaching this subject, so if you bring it up, that gives them permission. Physicians may need you to remind them of what is most important to the patient and to ask questions about whether their treatment recommendations will support your loved one's goals.

To improve communication between doctors, people with serious illnesses, and their caregivers, Ariadne Labs has developed a Serious Illness Conversation Guide. It encourages doctors to routinely ask their patients the following questions to establish a dialogue and help clarify end-of-life preferences.

- What is your understanding now of where you are with your illness?
- How much information would you like about what is likely to be ahead with your illness?
- What are your most important goals if your health situation worsens?
- What are your biggest fears and worries about the future with your health?
- What gives you strength as you think about the future with your illness?
- What abilities are so vital to your life that you can't imagine living without them?
- If you become sicker, how much are you willing to go through for the possibility of gaining more time?
- How much does your family know about your priorities and wishes?

Of course, caregivers and their families will have questions that they want to ask the doctor, too.

- What's the future for my loved one?
- What are the most important things I need to know as a caregiver?
- What kind of support is available for symptom control?
- How can I help keep my loved one from suffering?
- What can I do if my loved one is depressed?

Planning for palliative care

Palliative care, a multifaceted specialty aimed at improving quality of life, is a central part of treatment for life-threatening illness. It is not to be confused with hospice care, which is typically offered only when other treatments have been discontinued.

Palliative care can be administered at any time and at any stage of a person's illness—not just after curative treatments have stopped. It doesn't replace medical treatment; in fact, it is often used in conjunction with it to increase comfort and improve quality of life. Palliative care is useful in many serious illnesses—cancer, heart failure, Parkinson's disease, kidney failure, HIV/AIDS, amyotrophic lateral sclerosis (ALS), and chronic obstructive pulmonary disease (COPD), to name a few.

According to the National Institutes of Health's National Institute of Nursing Research (NINR), palliative care strives to provide

- expert treatment of pain and other symptoms—including shortness of breath, sleeplessness, nausea, depression, and loss of appetite
- open discussion about treatment choices
- emotional support for ill people and their families
- coordination of care.

Many patients who are considering palliative care wonder how their decision might affect their relationship with their doctors. The NINR offers the following clarifications:

- Your loved one does not give up his or her own doctor in order to get palliative care. The palliative care team and the doctor work together.
- Palliative care experts typically work closely with a person's entire medical team, including family doctors and specialists, nurses, and nutritionists.
- Most clinicians appreciate the extra time and information the palliative care team provides to their patients.

Research continues to show that palliative care offers real benefits to patients and their families. There is now clear evidence that palliative care helps control symptoms, improves patients' quality of life, and in some cases may help patients live longer. Yet many people feel that accepting palliative care means accepting that your loved one is dying. This is a misconception. The purpose of palliative care is to provide an extra layer of support for the patient and family in dealing with a life-threatening illness. It can be beneficial even if the person is ultimately cured, but it becomes increasingly important as people approach the end of life.

To locate a palliative care program near you, contact your loved one's hospital or go online to Get Palliative Care (https://getpalliativecare.org).

Hospice care

Once a word that evoked shelter for tired and ill religious pilgrims, the term hospice has come to describe a concept of end-of-life care centered on quality of life. Hospice care encompasses physical, emotional, social, and spiritual needs. When a cure is not possible and aggressive treatment isn't desired, hospice care offers symptom relief, pain control, and support. Such care may take place at home or at a nursing home, assisted living center, or hospice residence.

Hospice programs vary greatly but generally share certain characteristics:

A range of services. Hospice provides 24/7, on-call assistance. Hospice workers can visit the home, bring and administer pain medications, provide nursing care, supply durable medical equipment, and offer emotional support. Before and after a death, emotional support is extended to caregivers, too. Programs may offer bereavement counseling for a year after a death.

A multidisciplinary team. The hospice team typically includes specially trained doctors, nurses, home health aides, social workers, counselors, therapists, people who offer spiritual care, and volunteers.

Licensing, certification, and accreditation. Hospices must be licensed in most states. Those providing services covered by Medicare or Medicaid must also be certified by the Centers for Medicare and Medicaid Services.

Insurance coverage. Hospice services are covered nationwide under Medicare and in all states except Oklahoma under Medicaid, for anyone who has a prognosis of six months or less to live. Many private insurers also offer coverage. Hospice provides medications, medical equipment, and clinical services without additional cost to the patient.

Bereavement services. Certified hospices are required to offer bereavement services for family members of patients who die while in their care. Many also offer support groups and other bereavement resources for their communities.

The hospice team can work with you and your loved one to develop a personal plan of care. Family, partners, and close friends may be invited to help in many ways, such as by assisting with daily tasks like feeding and bathing and offering comfort by reading, sharing music, holding hands, and simply being present.

To locate a hospice program near you, ask a doctor for a referral or contact the Hospice Foundation of America (online at www.hospicefoundation.org or toll-free at 800-854-3402) or the National Hospice and Palliative Care Organization (online at www.nhpco.org or toll-free at 800-658-8898).

As you consider hospice programs, the Hospice Foundation of America suggests you ask whether each is licensed and Medicare- or Medicaid-certified, or certified by other organizations. Find out what services are available, whether insurance or Medicare or Medicaid covers these costs, and what out-of-pocket expenses are typical. Sometimes a sliding-scale payment plan is available for services that insurance will not cover. (Part of the basic agreement for hospice care is that the person will forgo life-prolonging treatments for the disease that seems likely to end his or her life. Medicare will pay to treat other diseases, however. And some insurers and some innovative hospice programs are willing to provide ongoing treatments for a life-limiting illness, under special circumstances. You should explore this with your insurer.)

It is wise to investigate hospice programs well in advance, so that you have an understanding of what they provide. Most hospices will offer an informational visit, to explain their services and how they would suit the patient. Consider what will be expected of you and whether the hospice's philosophy of care matches that of your loved one and other family members. And ask about support programs for caregivers and availability of inpatient services. Unfortunately, data show that many ill persons are admitted to hospice too late to reap most of its benefits. According to the National Hospice and Palliative Care Organization, more than a third of hospice patients die or are discharged within seven days of admission.

Sharing love and letting go

Preparing for the end of a loved one's life is one of the most challenging human tasks that we confront. Accepting that death may come—and then that it will come soon—requires tremendous strength. Sometimes family members worry that acknowledging this possibility will undermine their loved one's desire to live and continue fighting against the illness, or that it will make death come more quickly. However, most people find that preparing for a loved one's death, even while hoping that there will be more time, allows a sense of peace and facilitates coping with grief.

Although painful in so many ways, a serious illness offers you time to say "I love you," to share your appreciation, and to make amends. When death occurs unexpectedly, survivors often regret not having had a chance to do these things. Dr. Ira Byock, author of *Dying Well* and a longtime hospice advocate, suggests that people with serious illness and their families have conversations with each other that include four statements: "I love you," "I forgive you," "Forgive me," and "Thank you." Be specific. Express thanks for particular things. Talk about the times you've spent together that you will always treasure. If there have been wrongs on either side—and there usually have been—ask for and grant forgiveness.

Sometimes, people with serious illness and those who are dying hold on to life because they sense that others aren't ready to let them go. Family members should tell a dying person that it's all right to let go when he or she is ready to do so. The assurance that others will be able to carry on—perhaps to help children grow up or to fulfill another shared dream—may offer enormous relief.

Resources

Organizations

AARP
601 E St. NW
Washington, DC 20049
888-687-2277 (toll-free)
www.aarp.org

AARP is a nonprofit membership organization for people ages 50 and older. Its website offers many helpful publications on grief and end-of-life decisions.

CaringInfo (formerly Caring Connections)
National Hospice and Palliative Care Organization
1731 King St.
Alexandria, VA 22314
800-658-8898 (toll-free)
www.caringinfo.org

Caring Connections, a program established by the National Hospice and Palliative Care Organization, offers free information to people making decisions about end-of-life care. On the website, you'll also find articles on a variety of topics, including grief, advance care directives, caregiving, and hospice and palliative care. The website or toll-free help line can help you find a hospice or palliative care organization in your area.

The Compassionate Friends
900 Jorie Blvd., Suite 78
Oak Brook, IL 60523
877-969-0010 (toll-free)
www.compassionatefriends.org

This national nonprofit organization offers bereaved parents, grandparents, and siblings friendship and understanding delivered by others who have stood in their shoes. The website has a chat room and offers many supportive brochures for family members, friends, teachers, and various professionals.

Federal Trade Commission
Consumer Response Center
600 Pennsylvania Ave. NW
Washington, DC 20580
202-326-2222
877-FTC-HELP (877-382-4357, toll-free number for filing complaints)
www.ftc.gov

This government agency administers the federal Funeral Rule and offers an informative free brochure called "Shopping for Funeral Services."

GriefNet
P.O. Box 3272
Ann Arbor, MI 48106
www.griefnet.org

This online community offers email support groups for children and adults. The website also includes links to other helpful organizations.

Hospice Foundation of America
1710 Rhode Island Ave. NW
Washington, DC 20036
800-854-3402 (toll-free)
www.hospicefoundation.org

This nonprofit organization provides information on hospice services, publications on end-of-life decisions and grief, and links to local hospice agencies.

Additional websites

The Conversation Project
www.theconversationproject.org

This multimedia website focuses on helping people talk to loved ones and doctors about desires for end-of-life care.

Five Wishes
https://agingwithdignity.org/five-wishes

This is a national health care directive created by the nonprofit organization Aging With Dignity. Described as the "living will with a heart and soul," it includes questions to ask loved ones about care preferences, treatment, end-of-life decisions, and what they want loved ones to know. Five Wishes has been translated into many languages.

Podcast

Terrible, Thanks for Asking
https://www.apmpodcasts.org/ttfa

This podcast—also available through Apple Podcasts, Google Play Music, and iHeartRadio—consists of a series of interviews with people who've experienced different types of loss, including the death of loved ones. It is hosted by Nora McInerny, who suffered a miscarriage and the deaths of her father and her husband, all within the space of a few weeks.

Books about grief in children

Raising an Emotionally Healthy Child When a Parent Is Sick: A Harvard Medical School Book
Paula K. Rauch, M.D., and Anna C. Muriel, M.D., M.P.H.
(McGraw-Hill, 2006)

This practical, easy-to-read guide is a wonderful resource for families struggling with the dual challenge of raising children and dealing with a parent's illness. The practical advice offered in the book—such as reassuring the child that he or she will be taken care of, determining how children with different temperaments are truly feeling, and maintaining a daily routine and a sense of normalcy—comes from a program developed at Massachusetts General Hospital.

Understanding Grief in Children
Sharon Marshall Lockett
(Lockett Learning Systems, 2012)

This book examines how children grieve and how grief affects children at home and in school. It identifies signals that may indicate a child needs extra help in coping with a loss.